Gynaecology

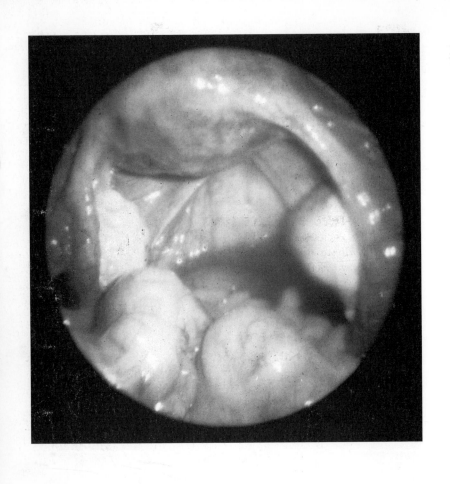

LECTURE NOTES ON

Gynaecology

GEOFFREY CHAMBERLAIN
MD, FRCS, FRCOG, FACOG
Professor of Obstetrics and Gynaecology
St. George's Hospital Medical School
London

JOHN MALVERN
BSc, FRCS (Edin), FRCOG
Consultant in Obstetrics and Gynaecology
Queen Charlotte's and Chelsea Hospital
London

FOREWORD BY
JOSEPHINE BARNES DBE

Seventh edition

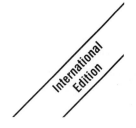

b
**Blackwell
Science**

*International
Edition*

© 1966, 1971, 1975, 1980, 1983, 1988, 1996 by
Blackwell Science Ltd
Editorial Offices:
Osney Mead, Oxford OX2 0EL
25 John Street, London WC1N 2BL
23 Ainslie Place, Edinburgh EH3 6AJ
238 Main Street, Cambridge
    Massachusetts 02142, USA
54 University Street, Carlton
    Victoria 3053, Australia

Other Editorial Offices:
Arnette Blackwell SA
  1, rue de Lille, 75007 Paris
  France

Blackwell Wissenschafts-Verlag GmbH
  Kurfürstendamm 57
  10707 Berlin, Germany

  Zehetnergasse 6
  A-1140 Wien
  Austria

First published 1966
Revised reprint 1969
Second edition 1971
Third edition 1975
Reprinted 1977, 1978
Fourth edition 1980
Fifth edition 1983
Reprinted 1984
Sixth edition 1988
Reprinted 1989, 1993
Seventh edition 1996
International Edition 1996

Set by Excel Typesetters, Hong Kong
Printed and bound in Great Britain
by Hartnolls Ltd, Bodmin, Cornwall

DISTRIBUTORS

Marston Book Services Ltd
PO Box 87
Oxford OX2 0DT
(*Orders:* Tel: 01865 791155
        Fax: 01865 791927
        Telex: 837515)

North America
Blackwell Science, Inc.
238 Main Street
Cambridge, MA 02142
(*Orders:* Tel: 800 215-1000
            617 876-7000
        Fax: 617 492-5263)

Australia
Blackwell Science Pty Ltd
54 University Street
Carlton, Victoria 3053
(*Orders:* Tel: 03 9347 0300
        Fax: 03 9349 3016)

A catalogue record for this title
is available from the British Library

ISBN 0-632-03111-5 (BSL)
ISBN 0-86542-816-6 (International Edition)

Library of Congress
Cataloging-in-Publication Data

Chamberlain, Geoffrey, 1930–
    Lecture notes on gynaecology/
    Geoffrey Chamberlain, John Malvern.
  —7th ed.
        p.   cm.
    Rev. ed. of: Lecture notes on
    gynaecology/Josephine Barnes,
Geoffrey Chamberlain. 6th ed. 1988.
    Includes bibliographical references
    and index.
    ISBN 0-632-03111-5
    1. Gynecology—Handbooks, manuals, etc.
    1. Malvern, John. II. Barnes, Josephine.
Lecture notes on gynaecology. III. Title.
    [DNLM: 1. Genital Diseases, Female.
    WP 140 C442L 1996]
RG110.C48 1996
618.1—dc20
DNLM/DLC
for Library of Congress   95-21884
                                              CIP

Contents

Foreword, vii

Preface to the seventh edition, viii

1 The gynaecological patient, 1

2 Clinical anatomy and embryology, 15

3 Physiology of the female genital tract, 47

4 The vulva and vagina, 57

5 The cervix, 71

6 The body of the uterus, 81

7 The fallopian tubes, 93

8 The ovaries, 103

9 Disorders of menstruation, 115

10 The menopause, 135

11 Sexually transmitted diseases, 143

12 Endometriosis, 151

13 Prolapse of the genital tract, 159

14 Urogynaecology, 173

15 Sexual problems, 183

16 Infertility, 193

17 Screening for gynaecological cancer, 209

18 Contraception, 217

19 Sterilization, 233

20 Termination of pregnancy, 241

21 Complications of early pregnancy, 249

22   The acute abdomen in gynaecology, 265

23   Gynaecological surgery, 277

24   Gynaecological epidemiology, 291

     Index, 303

Foreword

The year 1996 will represent the 30th anniversary of the publication of the first edition of *Lecture Notes on Gynaecology*.

I have always felt grateful to Blackwell Science for the invitation to write it. At that time I was actively engaged in teaching medical students and I was dismayed at the short amount of time allocated to obstetrics and gynaecology. This was largely because of the extension of their general syllabus with the addition of new specialities. This book is meant to provide a comprehensive account of the subject with clinical and scientific aspects.

Gynaecology remains an important part of medical education not only for those who intend to specialize but because those conditions which affect women in sickness and in health have a profound effect on their families.

The seventh edition as would be expected is a good deal larger than earlier ones: medical science is continually expanding and the frontiers of knowledge receding. Professor Chamberlain and Mr Malvern have produced a book which exceeds the intentions of earlier editions and should have the same appeal and success.

Josephine Barnes DBE
London

Preface to the seventh edition

The science of gynaecology is advancing rapidly. What was a basically clinical subject a decade ago has now forged a scientific infrastructure which is being enlarged yearly by basic reproductive research. Further, the humanization of medicine includes gynaecology and more consideration is now given for the women's ideas than was perhaps twenty years ago.

The three sub-specialities of gynaecology are now becoming full subjects to which scientists and clinicians are bending their attention. Reproductive medicine, urogynaecology and gynaecological oncology are practised by full time specialists in their field with research laboratories backing them up. Since Dame Josephine Barnes wrote the first edition of this book in 1966, the subject has exploded enormously, but the current authors have tried to keep the material inside the covers of a small book. This volume mimics the lecture notes of a retentive student who went to all the lectures and made full notes at all the tutorials. We have reduced the fine print and the hypotheses to a minimum and only hinted at research work in the offing; just enough to wet the appetite of those who may wish to specialize in this dynamic subject.

We have aimed to give a full cover of gynaecology for students preparing for the MB; the material, however, is a good basis for DRCOG students and also a beginning for those sitting the MRCOG Part II, especially if they come from overseas and are not familiar with UK clinical patterns.

Even with the enormous increase in material, Josephine Barnes' original ideas still come through the book. We hope that this symbiosis will go on linking classical gynaecology with the innovations that have come since.

Geoffrey Chamberlain
John Malvern
London

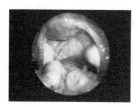

CHAPTER I

The gynaecological patient

History, 1
Examination, 4
  Abdominal examination, 4

Pelvic examination, 5
Examination with a
  speculum, 6

Bimanual examination, 7
Rectal examination, 8
Investigations, 8

Most women in the course of their lives will consult a doctor about gynaecological symptoms. Initially this will be with a general practitioner, for advice and maybe treatment. If the condition warrants, the woman may be referred to a hospital gynaecologist. Be it specialist or general practitioner, the same logical processes must be used to make a diagnosis.

The gynaecological assessment will be considered under three headings.

- History.
- Examination.
- Investigations.

HISTORY

This is best considered under systematic headings so that no important symptoms are omitted.

It is often necessary to ask leading questions.

- The woman herself may not realize the significance of her symptoms.
- She may be reluctant to mention symptoms connected with sexual troubles.

The following is a useful pro forma.

PERSONAL INFORMATION

- Name, age, date of birth.
- Married, single, widowed, divorced, separated.
- Occupation past and present.
- Hours and conditions of work.
- Partner's occupation.
- Type of housing.

CHIEF SYMPTOM

- Duration.
- Periodicity.
- Severity and description.

OBSTETRIC HISTORY

- Number of pregnancies.
- Dates.
- Mode of termination of each, i.e., full-term birth, premature birth, stillbirth, miscarriage, ectopic pregnancy.
- Abnormalities of:
    (a) pregnancy;
    (b) labour;
    (c) puerperium.
- Birth weights of children.
- Their present state of health.

MENSTRUATION

- Age at onset.
- Approximate duration of each period.
- Interval from the first day of one to the first day of the next.
- Estimate of amount and character of loss.
- Any recent change:
    (a) increase;
    (b) decrease;
    (c) clots in loss.
- Any pain associated with menstruation.
- Date of last period.

VAGINAL DISCHARGE

- Character of discharge:
    (a) mucoid;
    (b) purulent;
    (c) colour;
    (d) quantity;
    (e) bloodstained.
- Discharge may be offensive or may cause:
    (a) soreness;
    (b) irritation.

MICTURITION

- Frequency, day and night.
- Pain on micturition.

- Urge incontinence (micturition must occur on the urge).
- Stress incontinence (loss occurs on physical effort).

BOWELS
- Regularity.
- Use of purgatives.
- Any history of piles, pain or difficulty on defaecation.
- Rectal bleeding.

SEXUAL HISTORY
- Dyspareunia.
- Difficulty with coitus.
- Use of contraception.

HISTORY OF PAST MAJOR ILLNESS OR OPERATIONS
- All admissions to hospital with dates.
- A written report obtained from another hospital may be helpful especially with conditions such as infertility.

SOCIAL HISTORY
- Home conditions.
- Conditions of work.
- Occupation.
- Smoking habits.
- Alcohol habits.

FAMILY HISTORY
- Health of parents and siblings.
- History of hereditary or familial disease.

TREATMENT OF PRESENT COMPLAINT ATTEMPTED SO FAR
All drugs taken recently must be noted, especially tranquillizers, oral contraceptives, hormones and antibiotics.

The gynaecological history may be extremely simple where the complaint is straightforward.

The psychosomatic importance of history taking is determined by the patient being allowed time to explain her symptoms and feelings. The doctor can assess her character and whether she tends to exaggerate or underplay her complaints. Many women find it difficult to discuss the intimate and sexual details of their lives and so tact and discretion are needed. Further points of the history may come out during the physical examination.

EXAMINATION

The general appearance of the patient should be studied.
- Height.
- Overweight.
- Underweight.
- Does she look anxious or ill?

A systematic examination is made with special attention to the reproductive system.
- The lower eyelid mucous membrane should be inspected for anaemia.
- The breasts should be examined especially in the over 35-year-old.
- Other relevant symptoms, such as breathlessness or cough, call for examination of the heart and lungs.

Abdominal examination

The patient should be asked to empty her bladder before examining her abdomen and pelvis. The abdomen should be exposed from the costal margin to the pubes and the patient should lie comfortably relaxed. A sheet or light blanket over the pubis is used to prevent unnecessary exposure. The abdomen is inspected for:
- fat;
- wasting;
- striae gravidarum;
- distension;
- any visible tumour;
- operation scars (Fig. 1.1).

LIGHT PALPATION

This examination follows to test for any localized tenderness or rigidity.

DEEP PALPATION

Deep palpation is used to confirm the presence of a tumour or enlargement of:
- liver;
- spleen;
- kidneys;
- uterus;
- ovaries.

PERCUSSION

If there is a central tumour it will be dull to percussion with hollow sounds from the flanks. Ascites may produce shifting dullness in the flanks and central resonance.

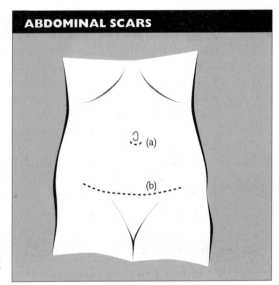

ABDOMINAL SCARS

Fig. 1.1 The two commonest abdominal scars used in gynaecology. (a) A laparoscopy scar, a crescent 2 cm long, below the umbilicus. (b) The Pfannenstiel or curved lower abdominal scar used for pelvic laparotomies.

AUSCULTATION

Although this will rarely help, it may give reassurance about intestinal activity, and bowel sounds may be heard. Fetal heart sounds may help make a diagnosis of pregnancy. Stethoscope auscultation after 25 weeks and handheld Dopplertone after 10 weeks.

Pelvic examination

THE VAGINA

Vaginal examination can almost always be satisfactorily performed by using the index finger alone. This causes less discomfort and muscle spasm. If the vagina is long or voluminous, a second finger may be needed, but this is in the minority of cases.

Assessment is by bimanual examination, the other hand being on the abdomen above the pubic symphysis. A three-dimensional image of the pelvis is built up from information obtained from both hands, not just the vaginal one (Fig. 1.2). Latex disposable gloves are best used.

THE VULVA

The vulva is inspected for:
- swelling;
- local soreness;
- inflammation;
- ulceration.

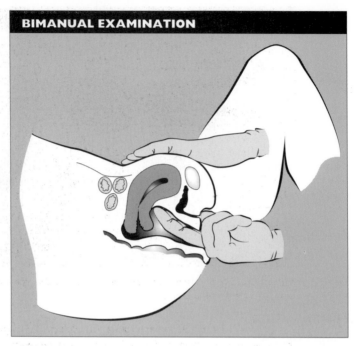

BIMANUAL EXAMINATION

Fig. 1.2 A bimanual examination gathers information about the pelvis with both hands.

THE URETHRA

The urethra is inspected for:

- urethritis;
- caruncle.

The patient is asked to cough or strain and any prolapse or stress incontinence of urine is noted.

Examination with a speculum

This is an essential part of the gynaecological examination. If it must be omitted because the vaginal entrance is too small or because of vaginismus, the examination is incomplete.

The *bivalve speculum* (Cusco's or Duck Bill) consists of two limbs jointed at the handle; it is made in various sizes and is useful for general cervical and upper vaginal examination. It is also made in a disposable plastic form (Fig. 1.3). A *Sim's speculum* holding back the posterior wall gives a good view of the cervix and anterior vaginal wall (Fig. 1.4). The *Ferguson's speculum* is a tube and gives good exposure of the cervix, but

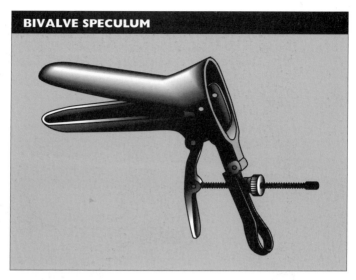

BIVALVE SPECULUM

Fig. 1.3 A bivalve or Cusco speculum used to examine the cervix with the woman in the dorsal position.

is rarely used in the UK. When passing a speculum, it is important to remember that the vagina is directed upwards and backwards; warming the instrument slightly in warm water makes the examination more comfortable for the patient.

Bimanual examination

When a cervical smear or a high vaginal swab is to be taken, it is best to pass the speculum before making a bimanual examination. This

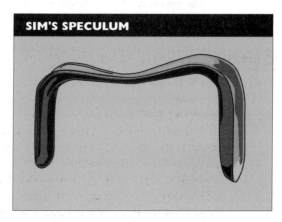

SIM'S SPECULUM

Fig. 1.4 A Sim's speculum used to hold back the posterior vaginal wall with the woman in the left lateral position.

examination may be performed in the dorsal or left lateral position, a matter of personal preference among gynaecologists. In either case the patient should be spared unnecessary exposure by covering her with a sheet or light blanket. The gloved index finger may be lightly lubricated and is introduced gently into the vagina.

- The condition of the vaginal walls is noted.
- The cervix is palpated for softening, tears or polypi.

The other hand is now placed on the lower abdomen and the uterus palpated between the two hands noting:

- size;
- consistency;
- shape;
- mobility;
- tumours;
- tenderness on pressure.

The finger in the vagina is now shifted into the right lateral fornix, the hand on the abdomen follows to explore for any enlargement or tenderness of the tubes or ovaries. A similar examination is made of the left adnexa. The finger is now passed into the posterior fornix to detect any swelling in the pouch of Douglas. The finger is then withdrawn and checked for any bleeding or discharge.

Rectal examination

This is often valuable in gynaecological practice, but the patient may find it the most uncomfortable part of the whole examination. It permits bimanual examination of the uterus, tubes and ovaries where vaginal examination is impossible or undesirable. It may further be easier to feel a retroverted uterus or a swelling in the pouch of Douglas. It allows an easier approach to the parametrium and utero-sacral ligaments, where the examiner may detect thickening due to infection, endometriosis or malignant growth in the parametria. The possibility of disease in the rectum itself must always be borne in mind.

INVESTIGATIONS

BLOOD

The haemoglobin level should always be measured before an operation, however minor. It should certainly be done in cases of menorrhagia, excessive uterine bleeding and as a routine in early pregnancy. Blood disorders may be associated with a bleeding tendency so a platelet count, bleeding time and clotting time may also be done.

In black women, a sickle test should be done and in women of Mediterranean or Middle East origin, there may be thalassaemia trait which is diagnosed by electrophoresis.

Serological tests of syphilis and HIV I antibodies are done if there is any suspicion of either disease.

The erythrocyte sedimentation rate is increased in chronic infections such as tuberculosis, in malignant disease, in pregnancy and in severe anaemia.

Blood urea and other tests for renal failure should be done where indicated.

Human chorionic gonadotrophin (hCG) levels in the urine may be checked if a pregnancy is suspected.

URINE

The urine should always be tested for albumin and sugar. Where renal tract infection is suspected, a mid-stream specimen is sent to the laboratory for microscopy and culture, after screening for bacilluria by dipstick. Further special tests, i.e., the white cell excretion, may be required in cases of chronic pyelonephritis.

CYTOLOGY

Exfoliative cytology in gynaecology examines cells desquamated from the epithelium of the genital tract. Material may be obtained by aspiration from the posterior vaginal fornix with a pipette, by scraping the cervix with Ayre's wooden spatula, or a micro brush or by scraping the vaginal walls. The following are among the uses of cytology.
• The early detection of premalignant lesions.
• Assessment of hormone secretion, oestrogens and progesterone and the determination of ovulation; it is a coarse study of endocrine disorders.
• Diagnosis and assessment of treatment in infections such as trichomonas vaginitis and in infection with vaginal thrush.

Cervical cytology may be used to diagnose non-invasive and micro-invasive carcinoma of the cervix; if every woman over the age of 25 had a regular cervical smear, carcinoma of the cervix could be abolished (Chapter 17). Malignant cells may be present in material obtained from the posterior vaginal fornix in carcinoma of the endometrium, fallopian tube and ovary, but this is unusual.

Colposcopy is a method of examining the cervix under magnification in the out-patient department. It is used in conjunction with cervical cytology so that biopsies can be accurately taken from suspicious areas.

OTHER PATHOLOGICAL INVESTIGATIONS

Hormones

Estimations of hormone levels in blood and urine may be required in a variety of conditions; they have wide ranges.

Histological examination of the endometrium

An important and useful investigation. Endometrium may be sampled in the out-patient department with a biopsy curette or Vabra aspirator. This allows histological examination of a sample of endometrium and may be sufficient for diagnostic purposes, for example in infertility. A full curettage permits a more complete examination of the contents of the uterus and is to be preferred in many cases.

IMAGING

Ultrasound

This is of value to detect and assess the consistency of pelvic tumours such as ovarian cysts or fibroids. A malignant cyst may be differentiated from a benign one by:

- An increased number of locules.
- Thickening of the tissue of partitions with solid areas.
- Disruption of the capsule.

With ultrasound, the size of the tumour may be estimated more accurately and the presence of tumours in the other ovary may be detected (Fig. 1.5). The vascularity of the tumour can be measured with Doppler ultrasound. Also fibroids can sometimes be detected and distinguished from ovarian cysts, a difficult clinical problem.

Ultrasound is used to monitor the progress of ovulation. A follicle can be found from day 10 of the cycle. Growth may be determined in a non-invasive manner by a daily scan. When the follicle reaches 20 mm it is just about ready for ovulation; this would be the best time for the harvesting of oocytes in an assisted fertility programme. After ovulation the Graafian follicle can be shown in the ovary.

Using ultrasound, the rare hydatidiform mole can be shown; the vesicles reflect echoes leaving a picture of a series of multiple semicircular reflections, rather like bubble foam lit from one side. There is usually no fetus present.

In early pregnancy, an embryonic sac may be seen by six weeks after the first day of the last menstrual period and embryonic tissue by seven

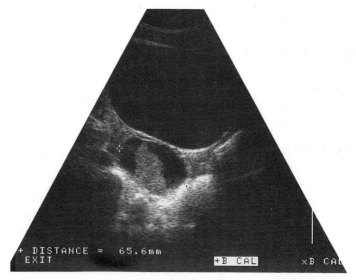

Fig. 1.5 An ultrasound scan of an ovarian tumour.

weeks. A blighted ovum can be detected if a sac is present but no fetus. The scan should be repeated a week later and if an empty sac still found, an evacuation performed.

Ultrasound is not of great help in the diagnosis of ectopic pregnancy. A woman admitted with low abdominal pain and vaginal bleeding may have a tender area in the pelvis; ultrasound may show this cystic area to be separate from the uterus but free blood in the pouch of Douglas is more predictive of an ectopic pregnancy. The presence of a sac *in utero* is reassuring, while if there is a positive pregnancy test and an empty uterus, this raises suspicion.

Magnetic resonance imaging (MRI)

If a very strong magnetic field is applied to the body, it polarizes the electrons spinning around every proton making up the hydrogen ion. If X-rays are now passed, energy is admitted to the radio-frequency from the displaced protons. In a series of measurements, cross-sections of the body can be clearly visualized since different tissues contain differing hydrogen ion concentrations.

Pelvic tumours are easily seen while tumour invasion from the endometrium, the cervix or from the ovary can be seen on different cross-sections, enabling staging of these growths to be made without an invasive operation (Fig. 1.6).

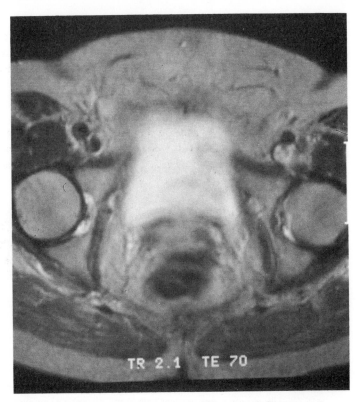

Fig. 1.6 An MRI scan of a pelvic tumour. With acknowledgement to Dr Christine Heron, Radiological Department, St George's Hospital.

Magnetic resonance equipment is currently available in few hospitals, but its use will spread.

Computerized tomography (CT) scans

These allow the visualization of many pelvic tumours to assess their position, size and consistency; it is much more readily available than MRI.

X-rays

Straight films of the abdomen can show gas and fluid levels in the intestine in obstruction. Furthermore, calcium in the urinary tract can be seen. Hysterosalpinography, with the injection of a radio-opaque fluid through the cervix, allows the outline of the uterine cavity and the fallopian tubes to be seen; as well as spill from the fimbriated ends indicating patency of the tubes at fertility investigations.

Intravenous urography

The diagnosis of pelvic tumours may be helped by intravenous urography, as well as cases where renal tract disease is suspected. It is usual to perform this investigation before radical operations in the pelvis such as Wertheim's hysterectomy.

Barium studies

A barium enema may be helpful in the differential diagnosis of rectal conditions and in the exclusion of a lesion in the colon. A barium meal with follow-through to the ileo-caecal region may be useful in cases where obscure symptoms are right-sided.

Pelvic lymphangiography

By injecting radio-opaque contrast material into the lymphatics in the leg, the lymphatic drainage of the lower limb and pelvis is outlined. It is useful to detect secondaries in the lymph glands from malignant disease in the pelvis.

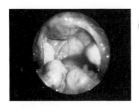

Clinical anatomy and embryology

The ovary, 15
  Structure of the ovary, 15
The fallopian tube, 19
  Structure of the fallopian tube, 19
The uterus, 20
  Structure of the uterus, 22
  Supports of the uterus, 25
The vagina, 26

Structure of the vagina, 26
The vulva, 27
The pelvic diaphragm, 28
The ureter, 31
  The course, 31
The bladder, 32
The urethra, 32
Pelvic arterial blood supply, 33
Pelvic venous drainage, 34

Pelvic lymphatic drainage, 35
Pelvic nerve supply, 36
Embryology of the pelvic organs, 38
Congenital malformations, 41
Chromosomes, 43
  Clinical conditions, 44
  Female sexual identity, 46

To the clinical student, anatomy may seem a subject finished with a few years ago. However, a working knowledge is required to understand the pathology and treatment of female genital diseases managed by gynaecologists.

THE OVARY

The ovaries have twin functions in both steroid production and gametogenesis. They are a pair of organs on each side of the uterus, in close relation to the fallopian tubes. Each ovary is attached to the back of the broad ligament by a peritoneal fold, the mesovarium, which carries the blood supply, lymphatic drainage and nerve supply of the ovary.

The ovary is a white wrinkled organ about the size of the end joint of a thumb. Its size varies but is approximately 4 cm long, 3 cm wide and 2 cm thick and weighs about 10 g. A general view of the organs in the pelvis is shown in Fig. 2.1.

Structure of the ovary

The ovary has an outer cortex and inner medulla (Fig. 2.2) and consists of large numbers of primordial oocytes supported by a connective tissue stroma. It is covered by a single layer of cubical, germinal epithelium which is often missing in adult women. Beneath is the fibrous capsule of

ORGANS OF THE PELVIS

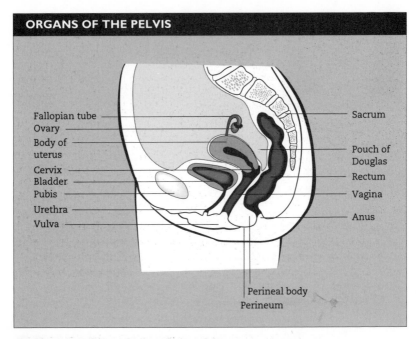

Fallopian tube
Ovary
Body of uterus
Cervix
Bladder
Pubis
Urethra
Vulva

Sacrum
Pouch of Douglas
Rectum
Vagina
Anus

Perineal body
Perineum

Fig. 2.1 A general view of organs in the pelvis.

FOLLICULAR MATURATION

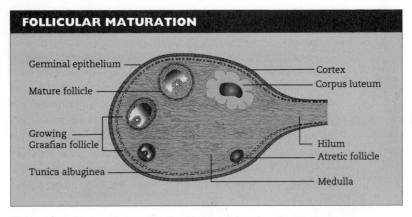

Germinal epithelium
Mature follicle

Growing
Graafian follicle

Tunica albuginea

Cortex
Corpus luteum

Hilum
Atretic follicle

Medulla

Fig. 2.2 Maturation of the oocytes to follicles.

the ovary, the tunica albuginea, a protective layer derived from fibrous connective tissue.

The cortex of the ovary at birth contains about two million primordial oocytes that may become follicles; cysts about 0.1 mm in diameter. They have a single layer of granulosa cells and specially differentiated stromal cells which secrete hormones.

MATURING GRAAFIAN FOLLICLE

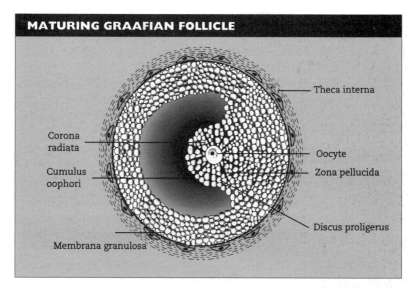

Fig. 2.3 Maturing Graafian follicle.

During each menstrual cycle many primordial follicles undergo ripening, but usually only one fully develops to become a Graafian follicle and expels its oocyte. The granulosa cells multiply and secrete follicular fluid. These push the oocyte, now 0.2 mm in diameter to one side. An oocyte is surrounded by a clear area, the zona pellucida and invested with granulosa cells, the corona radiata. The oocyte with its granulosa layer projects into the follicle (Fig. 2.3). The stroma cells outside the membrana granulosa differentiate into:

- the theca interna (hormone secretor);
- the theca externa (no hormone secreting function).

Shortly before ovulation, meiosis is completed in the primary oocyte. The oocyte casts off the first polar body resulting in the number of chromosomes in the remaining nucleus being reduced from 46 to 23. Thus the primary oocyte and the first polar body each contain the haploid number (23) of the chromosomes.

At this stage, the ripe follicle is about 20 mm in diameter. At ovulation it dehisces, releasing the oocyte with its corona radiata usually into the fimbriated end of the fallopian tube.

The follicle in the ovary collapses, the granulosa cells become luteal cells while the theca interna form the theca lutein cells. A corpus luteum develops and projects from the surface of the ovary. It can be recognized by the naked eye by its crinkled outline and yellow appearance. Its cells secrete oestrogen and progesterone. If the ovum is not fertilized, the corpus luteum degenerates in about 10 days. A small amount of bleeding occurs into its cavity, the cells undergo hyaline degeneration and a corpus albicans is formed. If pregnancy occurs, the corpus luteum grows and may reach 3 cm in diameter. It persists for 80 to 120 days and then gradually degenerates.

The ovaries of a 15-year-old girl contain some 500 000 oocytes, but by the age of 50 these are almost completely gone. Wastage of germ cells occurs by atresia at the time of ovulation each month and also goes as a continuous process from 15 to 50.

Many follicles mature but do not rupture and in these no corpus luteum is formed. In this case the fluid is gradually absorbed and the follicle regresses forming a small fibrous scar.

RELATIONS OF THE OVARY

The ovary lies free in the peritoneal cavity

Anterior	The broad ligament
Posterior	The peritoneum lining the posterior wall of the true pelvis The common iliac artery and vein The internal iliac (hypogastric) artery The ureter enters the pelvis in front of the bifurcation of the common iliac artery and is a close posterior relation
Lateral	Lateral wall of the pelvis with the obturator internus muscle The obturator vessels and nerve Further out is the floor of the acetabulum and the hip joint
Above	The fallopian tube The loops of bowel
On left	The pelvic colon and its mesentery
On right	The appendix if it dips into the pelvis
Fallopian tube	Curls over the ovary being in turn medial, superior and lateral to it

Box 2.1 Relations of the ovary.

The infundibulo-pelvic ligament is a double fold of peritoneum, continuous with the outer end of the broad ligament. It contains the ovarian vessels, lymphatics and nerves.

THE FALLOPIAN TUBE

The fallopian tube is embryologically part of the paramesonephric duct and continuous with the uterus. It is the oviduct conveying sperm from the uterus to the point of fertilization and ova from the ovary to the uterine cavity. Fertilization usually takes place in the outer part of the tube. It is in four parts.

- The *intramural* part is in the wall of the uterus. It is 2 cm long and 1 mm in diameter.
- The *isthmus* is thick-walled and lies near the uterus. It is 3 cm long and 0.7 to 1.0 mm in diameter.
- The *ampulla* is wide, thin-walled and curved, being about 5 cm long and 20 mm in diameter (Fig. 2.4).
- The *infundibulum* is the lateral end of the tube. It is trumpet shaped crowned with the fimbriae, frond-like processes that surround the outer opening of the tube. One fimbria is often longer than the others and is attached to the ovary, the fimbria ovarica. The fimbriae stabilize the abdominal ostium over the ripening follicle in the ovary. At the lateral end, it is 2 cm in diameter.

Structure of the fallopian tube

The tube has three coats.

- An outer *serous* layer of peritoneum which covers the tube except in its intramural part and over a small area over its attachment to the broad ligament.

RELATIONS OF THE FALLOPIAN TUBES

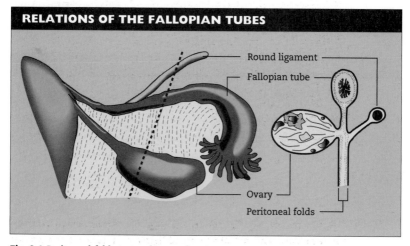

Round ligament

Fallopian tube

Ovary

Peritoneal folds

Fig. 2.4 Peritoneal folds to two layers of peritoneum.

• A *muscle* layer which in turn has outer longitudinal and inner circular layers of smooth muscle.
• The *inner mucosa* or endosalpinx which lines the tube that is thrown into numerous longitudinal folds or rugae. The rugae have a core of connective tissue covered with a tall columnar epithelium (Fig. 2.5).

Three types of cell are found in the mucosa.
• *Ciliated cells* which beat a current in a medial direction.
• *Secretory cells* which provide the secretion for the rapidly developing blastocyst allowing exchange of oxygen, nutrients and catabolites.
• *Intercalary cells* with long narrow nuclei, squeezed between the other cells. There are rhythmic changes in the epithelium during the menstrual cycle; in the proliferative phase the cells increase in height and activity with mural secretions just after ovulation.

RELATIONS OF THE FALLOPIAN TUBE

Anterior	Top of the bladder Utero-vesical peritoneal pouch
Superior	Coils of intestine Caecum on the right Pelvic colon on the left
Posterior	Ovary Pouch of Douglas and its contents
Lateral	Peritoneum covering the obturator internus muscle Obturator vessels and nerve
Inferior	Structures contained within the layers of the broad liagament

Box 2.2 Relations of the fallopian tube.

THE UTERUS

The uterus (Fig. 2.6) is a hollow muscular organ which lies in the centre of the true pelvis. It is mostly covered with peritoneum. Figure 2.7 shows the parts of the uterus.
1 The fundus is above the opening of the fallopian tubes.
2 The cornu is the angle into which each of the fallopian tubes opens.
3 The body makes up the main part of the cavity.
4 The isthmus is the narrow lowest part of the body between the histological internal os and the anatomical internal os.
5 The cervix is the neck which opens into the vagina.

The nulliparous organ is about 9 cm long, 6 cm wide and 3 cm thick, weighing about 50 g.

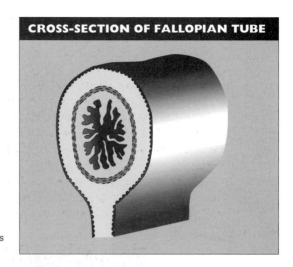

CROSS-SECTION OF FALLOPIAN TUBE

Fig. 2.5 Cross-section of the fallopian tube near its lateral end.

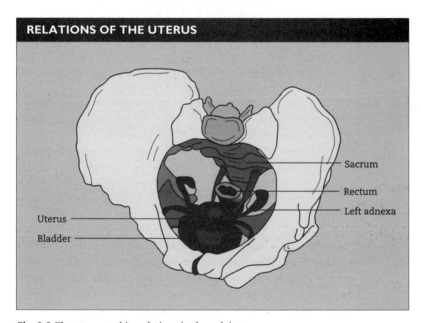

RELATIONS OF THE UTERUS

Sacrum

Rectum

Left adnexa

Uterus

Bladder

Fig. 2.6 The uterus and its relations in the pelvis.

In childhood the cervix exceeds the body in length. At puberty there is growth of the muscle so that the uterus becomes longer than the cervix. After childbirth the uterus is larger. At menopause and after, the body of the uterus atrophies to a varying degree.

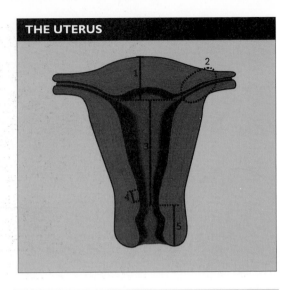

THE UTERUS

Fig. 2.7 The uterus.

Structure of the uterus

The body and fundus of the uterus are covered with peritoneum except at the sides, between the two layers of the broad ligaments. There are two layers of smooth muscle in the myometrium:
- a thin outer longitudinal layer continuous with that of the fallopian tube and the vagina;
- an inner layer arranged in oblique spirals (Fig. 2.8).

The epithelium is the endometrium and rests directly on the muscle with no intervening submucous layer.

The isthmus, 5 mm long, is lined by endometrium which is less sensitive to hormone influences. It becomes much larger in the pregnant uterus and forms the lower segment of the uterus in late pregnancy.

The cervix is a fusiform canal, a third of which lies above the attachment of the vagina with two-thirds projecting into the vagina. It is made mainly of fibrous and elastic tissue; the upper part contains smooth muscle which is condensed into a circular sphincter, the internal os of the uterus. There is a less constant external sphincter in the nulliparous woman (Fig. 2.9).

The cervical canal is lined by columnar epithelium, which has longitudinal folds and numerous oblique folds. The canal is lined by compound racemose glands which dip deep into the stroma of the cervix; these glands produce cervical mucous.

The vaginal part of the cervix is covered with stratified squamous epithelium continuous with that of the vagina. The junction between the columnar and squamous epithelium is at the external os in a nulliparous woman.

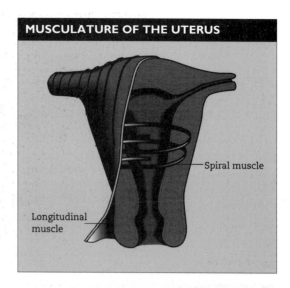

Fig. 2.8 The musculature of the uterus.

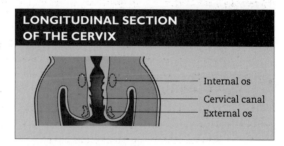

Fig. 2.9 A longitudinal section of the cervix.

RELATIONS OF THE UTERUS

Peritoneum	The body and fundus are covered with peritoneum
	In front, this is reflected and loosely attached to the upper surface of the bladder at the level of the internal os
	Over the rest of the uterus, the attachment is dense and it cannot be stripped off the uterine muscle
Anterior	The utero-vesical pouch and bladder
Lateral	The broad ligaments with their contents
Posterior	The pouch of Douglas
	The rectum

Box 2.3 Relations of the uterus.

RELATIONS OF THE CERVIX

Above the attachment to the vagina

Anterior	Loose connective tissue
	Bladder
	Pubo-cervical ligaments running forward to the back of the pubis
Lateral	The ureter lies lateral to the cervix 0.5 to 1 cm away from it
	The uterine artery dividing into:
	(a) ascending branches supplying the main uterus;
	(b) descending branches supplying the cervix and upper vagina.
	Uterine veins
	Parametrial lymph glands
	Nerve ganglia
	The transverse cervical ligament springing from the lateral side of the cervix and vaginal fornix
Posterior	Peritoneum, forming the anterior surface of the pouch of Douglas
	The utero-sacral folds from the back of the cervix, encircling the rectum, to the front of the sacrum

Box 2.4(a) Relations of the cervix above the attachment to the vagina.

RELATIONS OF THE CERVIX

Below the attachment to the vagina

The cervix projects into the vagina forming the four fornices

Anterior fornix	Separates the cervix from the vaginal wall and the base of the bladder
Lateral fornices	Separates the cervix from the vaginal wall to which are attached the transverse cervical ligaments
Posterior fornix	Separates the cervix from the pouch of Douglas and its contents. This is usually the deepest fornix

Box 2.4(b) Vaginal relations of the cervix.

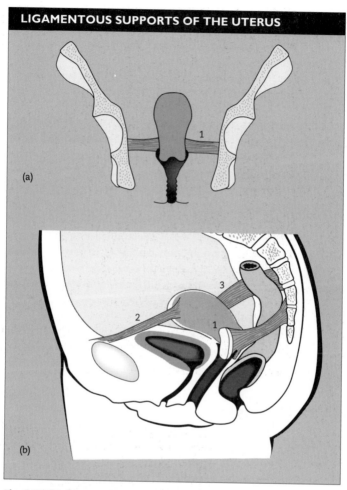

Fig. 2.10 The ligamentous supports of the uterus. (a) Frontal view. (b) Lateral view. 1. Cardinal ligaments. 2. Round ligaments. 3. Utero-sacral ligaments.

Supports of the uterus

The chief ligaments of the uterus are seen in Fig. 2.10.

1 Transverse cervical ligaments (cardinal) attached to the supra-vaginal cervix allowing the fundus of the uterus to be mobile so that it can expand, rising into the abdomen during pregnancy. These ligaments sweep laterally to be attached over the pectineal muscles on the side of the pelvis.

2 The round ligaments hold the fundus of the uterus forward but do not support it.

3 The utero-sacral ligaments running from the cervix to the lower sacrum.

The broad ligaments do not support the organ for they are only folds of peritoneum.

THE VAGINA

The vagina is a fibro-muscular canal extending from the vestibule of the vulva to the cervix, around which it is attached to form the fornices.

Structure of the Vagina

The anterior vaginal wall is about 10 cm long and the posterior wall 15 cm. It is capable of great distension, as in childbirth, after the prolonged hormonal stimulation of pregnancy. Normally, the anterior and posterior walls are in contact so the cavity is represented by an H-shaped slit (Fig. 2.11).

The walls have:
• an outer connective tissue layer to which the ligaments are attached—it contains blood vessels, lymphatics and nerves;
• a muscular layer consisting of an outer longitudinal layer and an inner circular layer of variable thickness and function;
• the epithelium of stratified squamous epithelium which in adult women contains glycogen and is composed of three layers:
  (a) a basal layer;
  (b) a functional layer;
  (c) a cornified layer.

The epithelium undergoes cyclical changes during the menstrual cycle and characteristic changes during pregnancy. After the menopause it atrophies so that smears taken from postmenopausal women contain a high proportion of basal cells. There are no glandular cells in the vaginal epithelium and so the term vaginal mucosa should not be used.

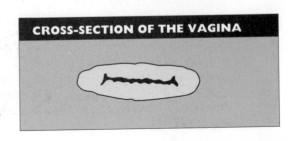

CROSS-SECTION OF THE VAGINA

Fig. 2.11 The vagina is closed fore and aft in the non-pregnant state.

Vaginal fluid in adult women is acid (pH 4 to 5). It is composed of cervical secretion and transudation through the vaginal epithelium. The vagina allows colonization of Doderlein's bacilli, lactobacilli which produces lactic acid from the glycogen in the epithelial cells.

RELATIONS OF THE VAGINA	
Anterior	The bladder and urethra
Posterior	Upper–the pouch of Douglas Lower–the rectum, separated by the recto-vaginal septum and perineal body
Lateral	The cardinal ligaments and the levator ani muscles

Box 2.5 Relations of the vagina.

THE VULVA

The vulva or external genitalia of the female includes the mons, the labia major, the clitoris, the labia minor, the vestibule, the external urethra meatus, the glands of Bartholin and the hymen (Fig. 2.12).

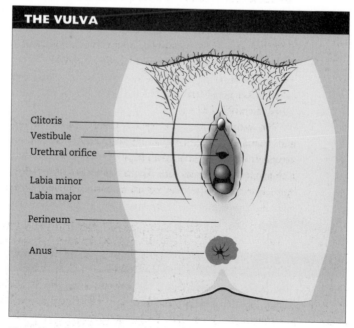

THE VULVA

Fig. 2.12 The vulva.

The *mons* is a pad of fat which lies over the pubic symphysis. It is covered with skin in which hair grows profusely from puberty to the menopause.

The *labia major* are two folds of skin which enclose the vaginal opening. They are made up of fatty tissue very sensitive to oestrogen stimulation; the skin of the labia major are covered with hair after puberty.

The *clitoris* contains erectile tissue and is attached to the pubic arch by its crura. Folds of skin running forwards from the labia minor form the prepuce of the clitoris.

The *labia minor* are delicate folds of skin, containing fibrous tissue and numerous blood vessels and erectile tissue. The skin contains sebaceous glands, but no hair follicles, and epithelium which lines the vestibule and vagina.

The *vestibule* is the area between the labia minor into which opens the vagina, with the external meatus of the urethra in front and the ducts of the Bartholin glands behind.

The *external urethral meatus* is the opening of the urethra covered with squamous epithelium. Skene's ducts from the posterior urethral glands open on to the posterior margin of the meatus.

The *Bartholin glands* are a pair of compound racemose glands, the ducts of which are lined by columnar epithelium. Each gland is the size of a pea and in structure resembles salivary glands. The glands are embedded in the posterior part of the bulb of the vestibule, a mass of erectile tissue lying in each labium minus. The duct is about 2 cm long and opens into the vestibule at the junction of the labium minor and the hymen between the anterior two-thirds and posterior one-third. The secretion is colourless and mucoid and is produced mainly on sexual excitement.

The *hymen* is a circular or crescentic fold of squamous epithelium and connective tissue which partly closes the vaginal entrance in young women. Its shape and size varies. It is often ruptured or stretched by tampon insertion or by intercourse—childbirth destroys it. Tags of remaining tissue are known as *carunculae myrtiformes*; these are of no practical use but act as a landmark for gynaecological surgery of the posterior vaginal wall.

THE PELVIC DIAPHRAGM

The pelvic diaphragm (Fig. 2.13) is made of the muscle and connective tissue which partly closes the spaces between the pelvic bones and supports the pelvic organs. It consists of:

THE PELVIC DIAPHRAGM IN CROSS-SECTION

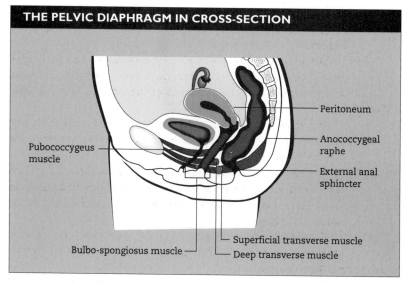

Pubococcygeus muscle

Peritoneum

Anococcygeal raphe

External anal sphincter

Bulbo-spongiosus muscle

Superficial transverse muscle
Deep transverse muscle

Fig. 2.13 The pelvic diaphragm.

THE PELVIC FASCIA

A thick layer lying on top of the levator ani muscle on each side. This is continuous laterally with the fascia covering the obturator internus muscle and medially with the fascial sheaths of the various pelvic organs.

THE CONNECTIVE TISSUE

These condense to form ligaments containing smooth muscle fibres, collagen fibres and elastic tissue. The main ones are:

1 the cardinal or transverse cervical ligaments running from the lateral pelvic wall to the supra-vaginal cervix and lateral vaginal fornix;

2 the pubo-cervical ligament running from the back of the pubic symphysis to the anterior part of the supra-vaginal cervix;

3 the utero-sacral ligaments running from the sacrum to the back of the supra-vaginal cervix and posterior vaginal fornix.

MUSCLES

The levatores ani are the principal muscles of the pelvic diaphragm. They consist of three parts.

- Pubo-coccygeus.
- Ilio-coccygeus.
- Ischio-coccygeus.

THE MUSCULAR PELVIC DIAPHRAGM FROM ABOVE

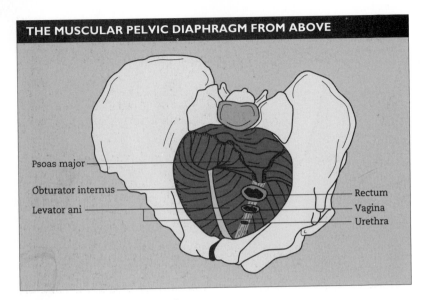

Fig. 2.14 The muscular pelvic diaphragm.

This sheet of muscle surrounds the vagina and supports the bladder (Fig. 2.14). Some of its fibres are inserted medially into the vaginal wall, the perineal body and the rectum. The triangular ligament or urogenital diaphragm consists of three layers shown in Fig. 2.15.

- Upper—the superior fascia of the levator ani.
- Middle—the deep transverse perineal muscle and compressor urethrae.
- Lower—the inferior fascia.

PERINEAL BODY

The perineal body is a pyramidal mass of fibro-muscular tissue into which are inserted fibres of the levator ani, the deep transverse perineal muscle, the superficial perineal muscles and the bulbo-cavernosus, but not the ischio-cavernosus.

SUPERFICIAL MUSCLES

The superficial perineal muscles consist of four muscles arising from each side.

- The *bulbo-cavernosus* or sphincter of the vagina passes from the perineal body, encircling the vaginal orifice to the erectile tissue of the bulb of the vestibule.
- The *ischio-cavernosus* runs from the lower border of the ischium to the bulb of the vestibule.

THE PERINEAL MUSCLES

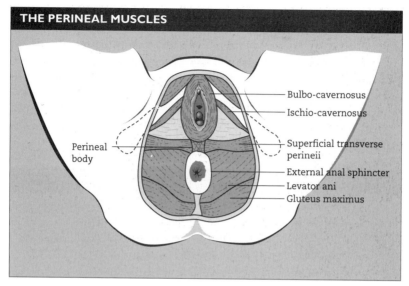

Bulbo-cavernosus

Ischio-cavernosus

Perineal body

Superficial transverse perineii

External anal sphincter

Levator ani

Gluteus maximus

Fig. 2.15 Peritoneal muscles of the pelvis.

- The *superficial transverse perineal* muscle originates in the perineal body laterally and is inserted into the posterior part of the ischio-pubic ramus.
- The *external sphincter of the anus* also arises from the perineal body. It has two parts:

    (a) the more superficial part spreads around the anus to be inserted into the coccyx;

    (b) the deep part encircles the anal canal.

The superficial perineal muscles are covered with a layer of deep fascia which separates them from the superficial fascia and the skin on the perineal area.

THE URETER

The ureter is a hollow muscular tube lined by transitional epithelium; the smooth muscle propels the urine from the renal pelvis to the bladder by peristalsis.

The course

The ureter is adherent and closely related to the peritoneum; it enters the pelvis passing in front of the bifurcation of the common iliac artery which lies directly in front of the sacro-iliac joint. The ovarian vessels cross in front of the ureter; on the left it lies behind the pelvic mesocolon. The tube passes down to the pelvic floor, lying anteriorly to the internal iliac vessels. At the pelvic floor, the ureter turns forward and medially, lying lateral to the rectum and entering the lateral ligament of the rectum. Then it passes through the transverse cervical ligament where it lies about 1 cm from the cervix at the level of the internal os. It next enters a fascial sheath continuous with the fascia covering the bladder and enters the bladder. In the pelvis the ureter receives its blood supply from a wide anastomosis fed by the internal iliac, uterine and inferior vesical arteries.

THE BLADDER

The bladder is a hollow muscular stretchable organ which acts as a reservoir for urine.

The upper part or fundus is covered with peritoneum. The base of the bladder or trigone is a smooth triangular area into which the two ureters open on each side posteriorly, with the internal meatus of the urethra at the apex. The bladder is lined by transitional epithelium while its wall consists of a complicated arrangement of smooth muscle fibres covered with a loose layer of areolar tissue.

The blood supply to the bladder is derived from the superior and inferior vesical arteries and that of the urethra from the inferior vesical, vaginal and internal pudendal arteries. There is a plexus of veins which drain to the internal iliac veins. The nerve supply arises from the hypogastric plexus.

THE URETHRA

The female urethra corresponds with the membranous part of the male urethra. It is about 4 cm long in the adult and is anterior to the vagina.

It too is lined by transitional epithelium in the upper part which merges at the external meatus with the stratified squamous epithelium of the vulva. The epithelium is thrown into folds and there is a subepithelial venous plexus. The muscular layer consists of longitudinal interlacing smooth muscle fibres, continuous with the muscle of the bladder; there is no anatomical internal sphincter.

Decussating fibres from the bulbo-cavernosus and ischio-cavernosus muscles surround it to form the striated, voluntary sphincter. Just above this the urethra passes between the two pubo-rectalis muscles, the anterior and inner parts of the levator ani.

Simple tubular glands open into the urethra posteriorly, of which the most prominent are Skene's glands, just inside the external meatus.

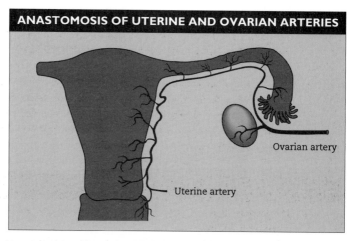

Fig. 2.16 Uterine and ovarian artery anastomosis.

PELVIC ARTERIAL BLOOD SUPPLY

THE OVARIAN ARTERY

This arises on each side from the aorta just below the renal artery. It runs on the posterior abdominal wall behind the peritoneum, crossing in front of the ureter and passing over the pelvic brim to enter the infundibulo-pelvic ligament. It supplies the ovary and enters the broad ligament to give branches to the fallopian tube and to anastomose with the ascending branches of the uterine artery (Fig. 2.16).

THE INTERNAL ILIAC ARTERY

This divides into an anterior and a posterior division (Fig. 2.17).
- *The anterior division*—continuous with the obliterated hypogastric artery, representing the umbilical artery in intra-uterine life. It generally gives off the superior and inferior vesical arteries, the uterine artery, the middle rectal artery and the inferior gluteal artery.
- *The posterior division*—gives off the ilio-lumbar artery, the lateral sacral arteries, superior and inferior, and the superior gluteal artery.

THE UTERINE ARTERY

A tortuous vessel running to the base of the uterus on each side at the level of the internal os. It gives off the cervical artery while the main vessel turns upwards between the layers of the broad ligament, giving a number of arcuate vessels which flow between the muscle fibres at right angles to the uterine axis. These terminate in numerous spiral arteries

THE INTERNAL ILIAC ARTERY

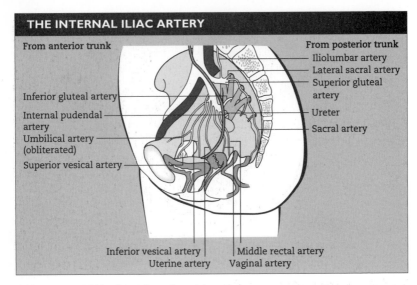

From anterior trunk

From posterior trunk
- Iliolumbar artery
- Lateral sacral artery
- Superior gluteal artery

Inferior gluteal artery

Internal pudendal artery

Umbilical artery (obliterated)

Superior vesical artery

- Ureter
- Sacral artery

Inferior vesical artery

Uterine artery

Middle rectal artery

Vaginal artery

Fig. 2.17 Arterial blood supply to the pelvis.

which supply the endometrium. In pregnancy some will become the placental bed arteries.

The main uterine artery passes on either side in the uterine substance to pass between the layers of the broad ligament just inferior to the fallopian tube. About a third of the way along the tube, the artery anastomoses with the branches of the ovarian artery.

THE VAGINAL ARTERY

This artery is a branch of the posterior trunk supplying the upper vagina.

THE INTERNAL PUDENDAL ARTERY

It leaves the pelvis through the sacro-sciatic notch supplying the vulva and lower part of the vagina, ending as the dorsal artery of the clitoris.

THE SUPERFICIAL AND DEEP PUDENDAL ARTERIES

These are branches of the femoral artery supplying the anterior part of the vulva.

PELVIC VENOUS DRAINAGE

The pelvic veins mainly correspond with the arteries and bear the same names. Extensive venous anastomoses exist around all the pelvic organs. The right ovarian vein drains into the inferior vena cava while the left drains into the left renal vein.

PELVIC LYMPHATIC DRAINAGE

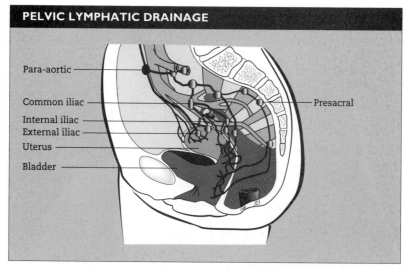

Para-aortic
Common iliac
Internal iliac
External iliac
Uterus
Bladder
Presacral

Fig. 2.18 Lymphatic drainage of the pelvis.

PELVIC LYMPHATIC DRAINAGE

The lymphatics of the ovary and fallopian tube drain with the blood vessels to the pre-aortic nodes (Fig. 2.18), a potential route of spread of cancer cells.

THE BODY OF THE UTERUS

The upper part of the body of the uterus drains with the ovarian vessels to the pre-aortic nodes. Its lower part drains to the broad ligament nodes and so to the pre-aortic nodes. From here drainage is to the para-aortic nodes. There is some variable drainage along the round ligaments to the inguinal nodes.

THE CERVIX

The cervix drains laterally to the nodes in the broad ligament, the internal iliac and obturator nodes: thence to the common and external iliac nodes. There is drainage along the utero-sacral ligaments to the pre-sacral lymph nodes.

THE VULVA

The vulva drains to both the superficial and deep inguinal lymph nodes and to the superficial and deep femoral nodes. There is some drainage direct to the internal and external iliac lymph nodes. The lymphatics of the vulva anastomose freely across the midline at the fourchette and the

PELVIC NERVES

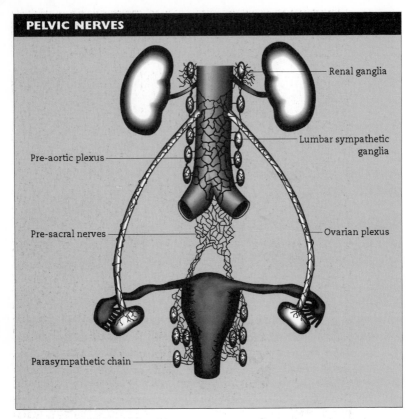

Renal ganglia

Lumbar sympathetic
ganglia

Pre-aortic plexus

Ovarian plexus

Pre-sacral nerves

Parasympathetic chain

Fig. 2.19 Nerves of the pelvis.

clitoral region. This is of importance in the spread of vulval cancer to the contralateral groups of lymph nodes.

THE VAGINA

Lymph from the upper part of the vagina drains with the cervix, from the lower part with the vulva.

PELVIC NERVE SUPPLY

The *fallopian* tube and the *ovary* are supplied by sympathetic and parasympathetic nerves which accompany the ovarian arteries (Fig. 2.19). The segmental representation is D 10 and 11 for the ovary and D 11 and 12 for the tube.

The *uterus* receives sympathetic nerves from the pre-sacral plexus which lies below the bifurcation of the abdominal aorta in front of the sacrum. The hypogastric nerve runs forward to the para-rectal plexus

THE PUDENDAL NERVE

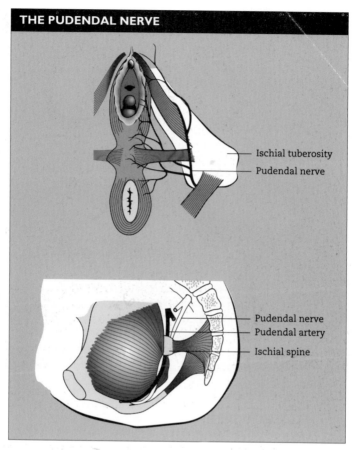

Ischial tuberosity
Pudendal nerve

Pudendal nerve
Pudendal artery
Ischial spine

Fig. 2.20 The pudendal nerve.

and the plexus in the base of the broad ligament. There are both motor and sensory nerves from D12 to L1. The pelvic plexus is joined by parasympathetic nerves, also motor and sensory from S2, 3 and 4.

The anterior part of the *vulva* is supplied by the ilio-inguinal nerve derived from L1 and the genito-femoral nerve derived from L1 and 2.

The remainder of the vulva is supplied by the pudendal nerve which is both motor and sensory and arises from S2, 3 and 4 (Fig. 2.20). This accompanies the internal pudendal artery into the pudendal canal; where it gives off the inferior rectal nerve which is distributed to the external anal sphincter, the lower part of the anal canal and the skin around the anus.

After leaving the pudendal canal, the dorsal nerve to the *clitoris* leaves. The rest of the nerve is the perineal nerve which supplies sensation to

DEVELOPMENT OF THE GENITAL TRACT

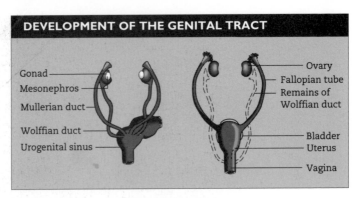

Fig. 2.21 Development of the genital tracts.

the labia major and minor, the perineum and the lower third of the vagina. It can be blocked with local anaesthetic injected into the pudendal canal—a pudendal block.

Muscular branches supply the superficial perineal muscles. The *levator ani*, the *coccygeus* and the *external sphincter ani* are supplied by muscular branches from the fourth sacral nerve.

EMBRYOLOGY OF THE PELVIC ORGANS

THE OVARY

Primitive germ cells arise from the endoderm of the yolk sac, developing in the genital ridge medial to the mesonephros high on the back wall of the abdomen. These germ cells are in the underlying mesoderm of the ridge with thickened coelomic epithelium over it (Fig. 2.21). All three make up the substance of the ovary.

The epithelium grows inwards to form a gonadal cord. The primitive germ cells multiply rapidly, until by 14 weeks of intrauterine life the female fetus has seven million primitive oocytes in each ovary. These reduce to two million by the time of delivery.

At this very early stage, the oocytes undergo prophase in the first division and remain thus until ovulation many years later.

The ovary is connected on each side to the uterus and thence to the inguinal fold by the gubernaculum. As the trunk grows, the ovary is pulled down towards the pelvis. The gubernaculum becomes secondarily attached to the uterus and becomes the ovarian suspensory ligament. The rest goes on to the inguinal region and becomes the round ligament which is usually attached at the caudal end to the pubic bone but may peter out into the labia major.

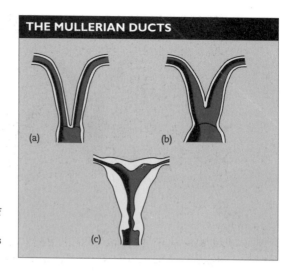

THE MULLERIAN DUCTS

(a)   (b)

(c)

Fig. 2.22 Development of the female genital tract from two Mullerian tubes (see text).

UTERUS AND TUBES (Fig. 2.22)

The Mullerian or paramesonephric duct (a) is lateral to the mesonephric duct and reaches the urogenital sinus at about nine weeks. The lower ends of the Mullerian ducts fuse (b) to form the uterus, cervix and upper part of the vagina (c), while the other parts remain separated as the fallopian tubes. Sometimes lack of fusion at the lower end of the Mullerian ducts leads to degrees of non-fusion uterine abnormalities.

VAGINA

The urogenital sinus grows inwards fusing with the bottom of the Mullerian ducts, which grow caudally. This is the vaginal plate at the junction of the upper two-thirds with the lower third of the vagina, the watershed of the lymphatic drainage. It is not the site of the hymen which is just below it. The vagina itself canalizes by 18 weeks of intrauterine life (Fig. 2.23).

Occasionally the vaginal plate is not fenestrated and the girl is left with an imperforate vagina behind which blood can accumulate when menstruation starts leading to a haematocolpos.

EXTERNAL GENITALIA

The cloaca divides into:
- an anterior urogenital sinus with the genital tubercle in front and genital folds on either side;
- a posterior proctodeum which joins up with the lowest point of the rectal cul-de-sac (Fig. 2.24).

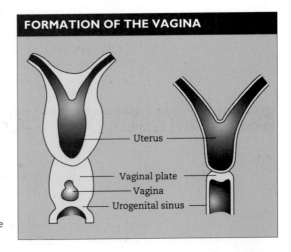

Fig. 2.23 Formation of the vagina.

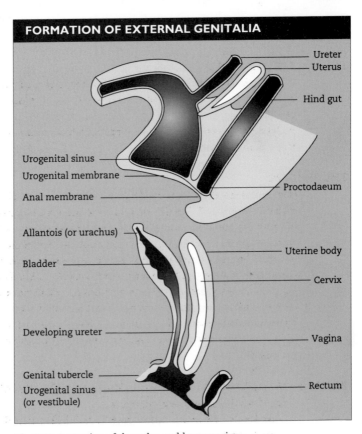

Fig. 2.24 Formation of the vulva and lower vagina.

By ten weeks gestation age:
- the front part of the urogenital sinus forms the urethra and bladder;
- the genital tubercle becomes the clitoris;
- the inner folds develop into the labia minor;
- the outer folds become the labia major.

CONGENITAL MALFORMATIONS

THE OVARY

- Agenesis of both ovaries—the uterus and vagina are present. This is Turner's syndrome where the chromosomal pattern is XO and so the individual is chromatin negative.
- Failure of development of one ovary is rare; it may occur in association with failure of development of the kidney, ureter and fallopian tube on that side.
- Accessory ovaries can occur along the line of descent of the gonad along the posterior abdominal wall in embryonic life.

THE FALLOPIAN TUBE

- Failed development in association with absence of a half uterus.
- Diverticula may occur in the tubes; these may predispose to ectopic pregnancy.
- Accessory ostea with a complete set of fimbria can be found on the antemesenteric border.

THE UTERUS

The uterus develops from the Mullerian ducts which usually fuse and become canalized. If they do not, it leads to uterine anomalies.

- *Aplasia of the uterus*—complete failure of development of Mullerian ducts so that the fallopian tubes, uterus and upper third of the vagina are absent. The vulva may be normal with a depression representing the lower part of the vagina. Primary amenorrhoea follows, but if the ovaries function normally, secondary sex characteristics will be normal.
- *Hypoplasia of the uterus*—may be a small fibrous nodule or hollow functionless sac, associated with primary amenorrhoea and may be mistaken for congenital absence. Primary amenorrhoea or scanty periods are usual.

FAILURE OF FUSION OF THE MULLERIAN DUCTS (Fig. 2.25)

The following degrees are encountered.

- *Anvil* uterus—the fundus fails to develop and the uterus is flat-topped.
- *Arcuate* uterus—there is a depression instead of a bulge at the fundus.

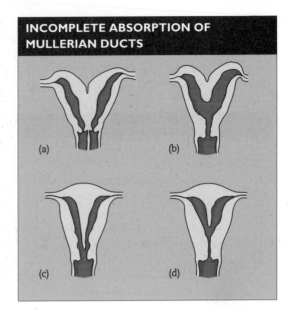

INCOMPLETE ABSORPTION OF MULLERIAN DUCTS

(a) (b)

(c) (d)

Fig. 2.25 Varying degrees of incomplete absorption of common walls. (a) Double uterus, double cervix, vagina septum. (b) Double uterus, single cervix. (c) Septate uterus. (d) Subseptate uterus.

- *Septate or subseptate* uterus—the uterus is outwardly normal but a septum, complete or partial, divides the cavity longitudinally.
- *Bicornuate* uterus—the lower parts of the ducts fuse, leaving two separate uterine horns. The cervix and vagina may be single or double.
- *Duplex* uterus or uterus didelphys—the two halves of the uterus are fully formed, each with its own cervix, often associated with division of the vagina into two by a septum.

Rudimentary uteri may be separated and have been described as far afield as in sacs of inguinal herniae.

THE VAGINA

A *longitudinal septum* in the vagina is often associated with imperfect fusion of the Mullerian ducts. It may be incomplete at the upper end of the vagina or complete coming down to the introitus.

Transverse septa may be found at the embryological junction of the Mullerian ducts and the urogenital sinus in the lower third of the vagina. They may be incomplete. A complete septum leads to cryptomenorrhoea and haematocolpos. The lower part of the vagina may be a solid cord; haematocolpos and haematometra may form above this.

The ureter may rarely open into the vagina. An ectopic ureter may open into the upper part of the vagina giving a continuous leak of urine from puberty, causing true incontinence. Remarkably, this is often not diagnosed until a girl is 10 to 13; at puberty there is a pelvic floor

NON-DISJUNCTION OF CHROMOSOMES

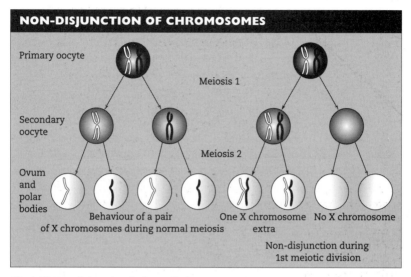

Primary oocyte

Meiosis 1

Secondary oocyte

Meiosis 2

Ovum and polar bodies

Behaviour of a pair of X chromosomes during normal meiosis

One X chromosome extra

No X chromosome

Non-disjunction during 1st meiotic division

Fig. 2.26 Non-disjunction during meiosis.

expansion and the girl may be brought to the doctor's for persistent bed wetting.

A pelvic kidney may be mistaken for an ovarian tumour.

CHROMOSOMES

The normal human has 46 chromosomes, 44 autosomes and two sex chromosomes. The number is halved in both gametes, the oocyte and spermatozoon; when fertilization occurs the original number is restored in the resulting fertilized ovum.

In the normal female the sex chromosomes are XX, in the normal male XY. All oocytes carry the X chromosome, while about half the spermatozoa carry X, the others Y. Thus, the resulting offspring are either XX (female) or XY (male).

Sex chromosomes abnormalities mainly arise from non-disjunction (Fig. 2.26). At the division of the primary oocyte while still sited in the ovary, the two chromosomes fail to separate so that a primary oocyte is produced which may have two X chromosomes or none; conversely, the first polar body will contain the converse—none or two. Fertilization by a spermatozoon which may carry X or Y can therefore result in abnormal patterns, XXX, XXY or XO. YO has not been described as this genetic combination is lethal.

The description is a simplification as more complex anomalies may occur, for example mosaics or individuals of mixed chromosomal pattern. Down's syndrome in its more common age-associated form results from non-disjunction of autosome number 21 resulting in trisomy 21; the rarer form is due to translocation of autosome 21 to another chromosome, usually 14. The latter is not age-associated and has a 50% chance of recurrence. Most Down's syndrome, however, is due to trisomy 21.

INVESTIGATION OF SEX CHROMOSOMES

Live cells can be taken from a buccal smear, a vaginal wall scrape, or the blood (maternal or fetal after 24 weeks) looking for sex chromatin. Chromatin positive cells are found in normal females, chromatin negative cells in normal males. The nuclei of the cells from a buccal smear contain a dark spot, the Barr body, when two X chromosomes are present (i.e. XX). Two Barr bodies indicate three X chromosomes (i.e. XXX).

Clinical conditions

TURNER'S SYNDROME
- Chromosome pattern XO.
- Incidence about 3 in 10000 full-term births.
- Present with primary amenorrhoea for there are either no ovaries or non-functioning streaks of tissue with no oogenesis.
- The vagina and uterus are present.
- Poor breast development.
- Little or no axillary and pubic hair.
- Short stature.
- Webbing of the neck.
- A wide carrying angle in the arms.
- Coarctation of the aorta.
- Congenital malformation of the kidneys may be found.

SUPER FEMALES
- Chromosomal pattern XXX or even XXXX.
- Usually secondary amenorrhoea and mental defect.
- These women are usually sterile but a few give birth to children.

KLINEFELTER'S SYNDROME
- Chromosomal pattern XXY.
- These are males who are exceptionally tall.
- Infertile.
- Eunuchoid.
- Small soft testes.

- May have gynaecomastia.
- Mental defect.

TESTICULAR FEMINIZATION
- Chromosomal pattern XY.
- May be either testicular feminization or androgen insensitivity.
- Active breast development.
- Absent or scanty axillary and pubic hair.
- May be absent uterus often with a very short vagina.
- The gonads are testes and may be intra-abdominal or in the labia major.

TRUE HERMAPHRODITES
- Occur with both ovarian and testicular tissues. Very rare.

THE ADRENO-GENITAL SYNDROME
- Chromosomal pattern XX.
- Congenital adrenal hyperplasia inherited as a Mendelian recessive.

SEXUAL IDENTITY

The development of female sexuality is closely linked to the physical and psychological changes attributable to the male or female

In infancy the baby girl is closely related to her mother who is the centre of her world. As she grows up she may become jealous of her parents' physical enjoyment of each other and may come to regard her mother as a madonna (in the old fashioned sense) or as a witch

As puberty approaches, the girl becomes aware of the physical changes in her body; to some the appearance of 'puppy fat' may be revolting and she may reject her femininity leading to anorexia nervosa which is most commonly seen in adolescent girls

At puberty her relationship with her mother may change and a phase of adolescent rebellion is common. This often coincides with the girl's first serious sexual encounter with a boy. She may have been told since infancy to regard the genital area as banned and if she embarks on a sexual relationship this may lead to guilt feelings

Most girls live through this phase to become mature women, to achieve normal sexual relationships and eventually marriage and childbearing. The girl's normal sexual development may be arrested, perhaps by over-protective parents so that she finds it difficult to achieve a satisfying relationship in adult life

Box 2.6 Sexual identity.

- Female infants are born with ambiguous genitalia.
- Defective production of cortisol, due to 21-hydroxylase deficiency.
- Leads to overproduction of corticotrophic hormone and enlargement of the adrenal cortex.
- The clitoris is enlarged and the labia fused.
- Some of these babies are salt losers and become seriously ill in the first week of life.

VIRILIZATION IN ADULT LIFE

May result from:

- The increased production of testosterone in the adrenal glands.
- Masculinizing tumour of the ovary such as an arrhenoblastoma.
- Polycystic ovarian disease.

Female sexual identity

Sexual identity can be at different levels. Box 2.6 outlines some of them.

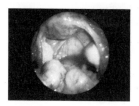

Physiology of the female genital tract

The ovary, 47
Major ovarian hormone
groups, 49
Oestrogens, 49
Progesterone, 50

Pituitary gonadotrophin
hormones, 50
Function of the organs, 51
The uterus, 51
The menstrual cycle, 51

The fallopian tubes, 55
The vulva and vagina, 56
Sexual activity, 56
Childbirth, 56

The functions of the female genital tract are to:
• act as a coordinated system to facilitate reproduction of the species;
• allow the embyro to develop to a mature stage *in utero* before being expelled;
• metabolize the hormones required in reproductive life.
    These functions are associated with:
• fertilization;
• maintenance of the pregnancy;
• expulsion of the baby at full term;
• hormone production for:
    (a) sexual drive;
    (b) effect it has on total metabolism.

THE OVARY

In each menstrual cycle over 400 primitive oocytes migrate to the surface of the ovaries. One or two of these attenuate the layers of follicle which become ischaemic (Fig. 3.1). When one follicle reaches 20mm in diameter, the oocyte and follicular fluid are squeezed out onto the surface of the ovary. The remaining follicles become atretic.
    The process of ovulation is preceded by:
• the release of luteinizing hormone (LH) from the pituitary which initiates ovulation;
• a spurt of oestrogen from the tissues of the follicle.
    The oocyte is oozed into the fimbrial end of the fallopian tube. Fertilization by the spermatozoon takes place in the lateral third of the tube. Sperm penetration initiates the second meiotic division of the ovum, with a reduction in chromosomes from 46 to 23 and the extrusion

THE FOLLICLE AND OOCYTE RELEASE

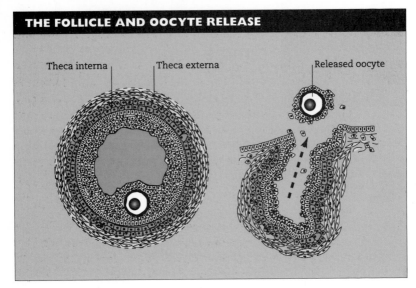

Theca interna   Theca externa   Released oocyte

Fig. 3.1 The follicle just before and just after the oocyte is released.

of a second polar body. Fertilization with the sperm results in the reconstitution of the diploid state — 46 chromosomes.

The signs and changes associated with ovulation are:
• the cervical mucus becomes less viscid and increases in amount;
• occasionally slight bleeding from the endometrium — in some women peritoneal pain is caused by irritation of released blood from the follicle (mittelschmerz);
• the basal body temperature may increase by about 0.6°C caused by the pyrogenic affect of progesterone.

GERM CELLS

There are about seven million primordial oocytes or germ cells in each ovary of the female fetus at 15 weeks of intrauterine life. This drops to two million germ cells at birth and is further reduced to half a million at puberty.

About 400 will be released during each ovulation cycle during the reproductive life; the rest degenerate at a steady rate. At the menopause there are no more follicles available for ovulation and so there is diminution of oestrogen production. The stromal tissue of the ovary produces androgenic hormones which may be metabolized in peripheral fat to produce oestrogens.

Ovulation is controlled by the ovarian hormones and the gonadotrophins from the pituitary.

MAJOR OVARIAN HORMONE GROUPS

Oestrogens

These are produced by the maturing follicle and in the ovarian stroma. Other sites are the adrenal glands and the subcutaneous fat layer. Levels gradually increase to a peak at the time of ovulation. Oestrogens occur in several forms (Fig. 3.2).

- Oestradiol—the active form; the major hormone in the human.
- Oestriol—less active, but produced in large amounts during pregnancy.
- Oestrone—relatively inert and the most prominent after the menopause.

The recognized functions of oestrogens are to:

- stimulate growth of the vagina, uterus and oviducts in puberty;
- increase the thickness of the vaginal wall and distal one third of the urethra by increased stratification of the epithelium;
- increase glycogen content in the cells of the vaginal wall;
- reduce vaginal pH by the action of the Doderlein's bacillus on the glycogen to form lactic acid;
- decrease the viscosity of cervical mucus;
- facilitate the development of primordial follicles;
- inhibit follicle stimulating hormone (FSH) secretion;
- stimulate proliferation of the endometrium;

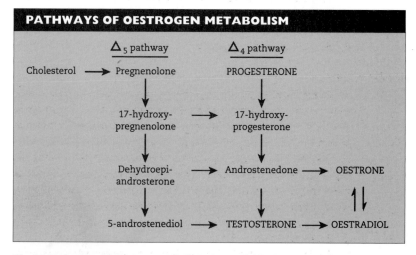

Fig. 3.2 Pathways of oestrogen metabolism. Oestradiol is a pregnancy oestrogen metabolized by the fetoplacental unit and does not appear here.

- increase myometrial contractility;
- stimulate growth of breasts with duct proliferation;
- promote calcification of bone;
- promote female fat distribution;
- promote female hair distribution.

Oestrogen is metabolized by the liver and conjugated with glucuronic acid:

- 65% is excreted in urine;
- 10% is excreted in faeces;
- 25% is metabolized in other substances.

Progesterone

This hormone is produced by the corpus luteum in large amounts following ovulation and by the placenta in pregnancy. Its functions are to:

- induce secretory changes in the endometrium previously prepared by higher oestrogen levels;
- increase the viscosity of cervical mucus;
- increase the growth of the myometrium in pregnancy;
- decrease myometrial activity in pregnancy;
- increase secretory activity in the fallopian tubes;
- decrease motility of the fallopian tubes;
- increase the glandular areas of the breasts;
- increase the sebaceous secretion activities throughout the body—premenstrual acne in puberty may follow unbalanced progesterone secretion.

Progesterones are metabolized:

- 80% is changed to pregnanediol in the liver;
- 20% is excreted in the urine.

Pituitary gonadotrophin hormones

FOLLICULAR STIMULATING HORMONES (FSH)

These are soluble glycoproteins. Production is activated by gonadotrophic releasing hormones (GnRH) from the hypothalamus. FSH is produced in the anterior lobe of the pituitary and production is increased in the first half of the menstrual cycle. This production is diminished by increasing oestrogen levels (negative feedback) (Fig. 3.3).

LUTEINIZING HORMONE (LH)

This is another soluble glycoprotein activated in the pituitary by GnRH. The luteinizing hormone is released from the pituitary as a

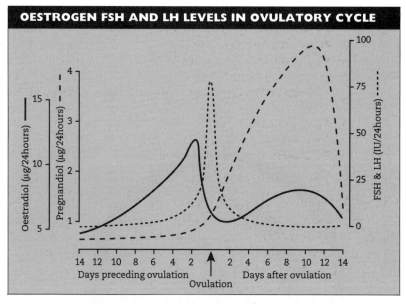

OESTROGEN FSH AND LH LEVELS IN OVULATORY CYCLE

Fig. 3.3 Hormone levels before and after ovulation.

bolus mid-cycle initiating ovulation if the follicle is already primed by oestrogen.

FUNCTION OF ORGANS

The uterus

The main functions are to:
- provide a site for placental implantation which will act as the exchange station of the embryo;
- provide a protection environment for the developing embyro;
- deliver the fetus after about 38 weeks of intrauterine life.

When fertilization of the embryo does not take place, the endometrium which has been prepared is shed about every four weeks from menarche to menopause as a menstrual period.

The menstrual cycle

The cyclical interaction of the hormones from the hypothalmus, anterior pituitary and the ovaries is shown in Fig. 3.4.
- The production of oestrogen and later both oestrogen and progester-

CYCLICAL INTERACTION OF HORMONES

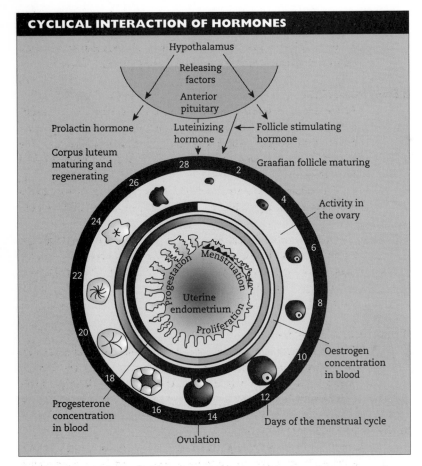

Fig. 3.4 Composite diagram of the menstrual cycle and histology of the endometrium.

one by the ovaries. This results in preparation changes in the endometrium lining the uterus.

• The *endometrium* is the mucous membrane of the uterus, consisting of tubular glands with supporting stroma. There are numerous blood vessels which arise from the spiral arterioles; the terminal branches of the uterine arteries.

• The endometrium rests on the *uterine musculature*; its basal areas are so closely applied they cannot be removed with a curette.

• The *basal layer* contains blind end tubular glands which regenerate following menstruation and childbirth. Unlike the superficial layers, the deep layer is less sensitive to hormonal influence and remains unchanged during the phases of the menstrual cycle.

- The *intermediate sponge layer* is a loose structure which separates when the endometrium is shed.
- The *superficial compact layer* is covered with ciliated columnar epithelial cells which extend down into the endometrial glands.

MENSTRUATION

At the end of menstruation the endometrium enters a short resting phase, when it is thin, its glands are straight and the stroma compact and non-vascular. Follicular stimulating and luteinizing hormone cause the maturation and growth of the follicles which results in higher secretion of oestrogen.

The endometrium enters a follicular or proliferative phase when the endometrial glands grow becoming tortuous; the stroma becomes more cellular.

After ovulation, the corpus luteum is formed under the influence of the luteinizing hormone; it secretes oestrogen and progesterone. In the luteal phase, the endometrium becomes secretory; it is thick, pale and glycogen appears in the glands which in turn become full of secretions.

If the ovum is fertilized

The endometrium continues to grow and becomes the decidua of pregnancy. The stroma cells swell and the glands become scarce. Implantation occurs on tissue, which is able to provide nutrition for the rapidly developing blastocyst.

In the absence of fertilization

About 14 days after ovulation there is an intense spasm of the endometrial arterioles leading to tissue hypoxia and death in the middle and superficial layers. Cracking and fissuring of the endometrium follows with cleavage of the endometrium from its spongy layer. It is shed in small areas with accompanying bleeding—the menstrual loss. Following this, regeneration occurs from the remaining basal layer and the cycle recommences.

THE MENSTRUAL FLOW (MENSES) CHARACTERISTICS

- Blood and desquamated endometrium with some added cervical mucus and vaginal cells in its passage down the lower genital tract.
- Usually there is no clotting of menstrual blood because fibrinolytic enzymes in the uterine cavity cause lysis. There is also some release of heparin from the mast cells of the endometrium. If there is more bleeding than is usual for that woman, menstrual blood then contains clots.

- The normal volume is approximately 50 ml; the range is 5 ml to 75 ml. More than 80 ml is considered to be abnormal loss.
- Heavy loss is associated with clots and cramping pains.
- There is a wide variation in the length of the menstrual cycle. The mean is 28 days with a variation of seven days.
- The duration of flow is approximately two to five days with the heaviest loss usually on day two and the last 24 to 48 hours being of darkened blood and brown discharge.

MEASUREMENT OF MENSTRUAL LOSS

- Directly by collecting loss in a series of cervical caps—difficult, cumbersome and inaccurate.
- Indirectly by lysing the haemoglobin out of all the collected menstrual pads with their loss—inelegant, but valid.
- Indirectly with radio-tagged red cells (Cr_{60}) to measure radioactivity.
- Practically—history of:
    (a) clots;
    (b) sharp change in pad usage.
- Practically—ask the woman to describe loss on pad in relation to coins (Fig. 3.5).

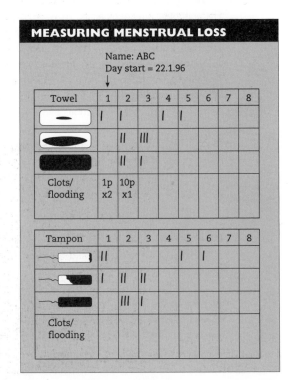

MEASURING MENSTRUAL LOSS

Name: ABC
Day start = 22.1.96

Towel	1	2	3	4	5	6	7	8
▬	I	I		I	I			
⬤		II	III					
▬		II	I					
Clots/ flooding	1p x2	10p x1						

Tampon	1	2	3	4	5	6	7	8
▭	II				I	I		
▭	I	II	II					
▭		III	I					
Clots/ flooding								

Fig. 3.5 Assessment of menstrual blood loss using the pictorial blood loss assessment chart. With acknowledgement to Dr J Higham. Brit J Obstet Gyn **97**, 734.

THE FALLOPIAN TUBES

Their functions are:

• to convey a spermatozoa from the endometrial cavity to the site of fertilization in the outer third of the fallopian tube;

• to transmit the fertilized oocyte from the fallopian tube into the endometrial cavity;

• to provide nutrients to the developing embryo on its five day passage.

Oestogen reduces the peristalsis of the tubes; at the time of ovulation there is a reversal to help the sperm to travel up more easily. The spermatozoa swim up the crypts between the folds of the mucous lining of the tube.

The oocyte is squeezed out of the follicle and sticks to the surface of the ovarian fimbria of the tube. The fimbria embraces the ovary and the oocyte moves directly into the fallopian tube without the need for transperitoneal journey. Fertilization is by a single sperm penetrating the zona pellucida (Fig. 3.6).

Peristalsis of the muscle of the tube and the action of the fine cilia moves oviduct fluid and the passive ovum from the peritoneal end of the fallopian tube into the endometrial cavity. This takes about five days.

During this passage, the fertilized ovum receives nutrition from secretions of the mucosa of the tube. Here gas exchange of oxygen and carbon dioxide between the rapidly growing blastocyst and fallopian tube fluid also takes place. These tubal secretions are under the influence of oestrogen priming and increase greatly with progesterone. Mucopolysaccharide concentration and the calcium ions within the tubes, which are essential for the functioning of the muscular cells, also increase.

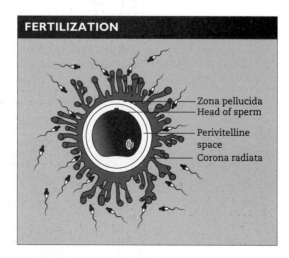

FERTILIZATION

Zona pellucida
Head of sperm
Perivitelline space
Corona radiata

Fig. 3.6 Several sperms surround the oocyte, but only one penetrates.

THE VULVA AND VAGINA

The vagina is a tube lined by stratified squamous epithelium which contains no mucous glands and thus there are no vaginal secretions. Any lubrication is a combination of secretions from the mucous glands at the cervical canal mixed with secretions from vulval glands and a transudate from the vagina.

The labia minor are normally in apposition; the fatter labia major are also together in normal standing, sitting and lying down positions.

Sexual activity

On sexual stimulation, there is a vascular engorgement of the labia major, minor and the clitoris. The sweat glands of the labia minor have increased secretions. Transudation across the vaginal wall is increased and at the same time mucus is secreted from the Bartholin's glands and endocervical glandular epithelium.

Abduction of the thighs opens the labia major and the voluntary musculature of the vagina and vulva help to dilate the upper vagina whilst gripping the penis in the lower vagina.

The sexual response in women is usually slower than in men but a plateau of response is more prolonged and it does not disappear rapidly after orgasm as is often the case in men.

Childbirth

During pregnancy, oestrogen increases vascularity and progesterone permits muscular relaxation and softening of the connective tissue sheath of the vagina by an increase in fluid. In consequence, over 38 weeks the tube becomes much more stretchable so that by full term, the vagina and vulva permit the passage of an infant with a head diameter of approximately 10 cm. The perineum with the squamous epithelium in the region of the fourchette does not always stretch so readily in the crowning of the fetal head and so may tear on occasions.

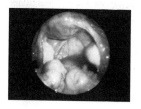

The vulva and vagina

The vulva, 57
  Pruritus vulvae, 57
Lump in the vulva, 59
  Conditions of the vulva, 59
Malignant disease of the vulva, 61
  Squamous epithelioma, 61

Adeno-acanthoma, 62
Intra-epithelial carcinoma, 63
Basal cell carcinoma, 63
Malignant melanoma, 63
The vagina, 63
  Infections of the lower genital tract, 63
  Microbiology, 65

Gardnerella, 65
Trichomonas, 66
Monilia (thrush), 67
Septic shock syndrome, 68
Atrophic vagina, 68
Foreign bodies in the vagina, 69

THE VULVA

The vulva is subject to:
- diseases which affect the skin in general;
- certain conditions specific to the vulva.

Pruritus vulvae

Pruritus vulvae is a common symptom—an irritation of the vulva sufficient to lead to scratching.

CAUSES

Irritating vaginal discharges of trichomonas vaginalis or monilia. Since many infections are common to the vulva and vagina, these are considered collectively in later sections. Other causes are varied.
- *Parasites* such as scabies and crab lice.
- *Fungi* such as athlete's foot affects the feet, the groin and the vulva.
- *Sensitivity to drugs* or chemicals including:
  (a) soap and disinfectants;
  (b) detergents used for washing underwear;
  (c) contraceptives made of rubber;
  (d) commercial spermicides;
  (e) ointments containing benzocaine and amethocaine.

- *Iron deficiency anaemia* associated with glossitis.
- *Gross vitamin deficiencies*, A and B group; especially in elderly women.
- *Glycosuria* due to any cause, but principally diabetes. Glycosuria probably causes irritation because the vulva becomes infected with a fungus. A glucose tolerance test must be done.

Degenerative conditions of the vulva occur mainly in postmenopausal women and are associated with irritation and soreness. There are two main varieties.

- *Leukoplakia of the vulva*—an important, but uncommon condition specific to the vulva. It presents as a thickening and hypertrophy of the vulval skin often spreading into the groin and around the anus. The hypertrophic keratin layer causes white patches; hence the name. It may be precancerous and tends to recur in time after surgical removal of the vulva. Diagnosis is by biopsy; this shows thickening and increase in depth of the keratin layer, while the basal papillae are hypertrophied and dip deeply into the corium.
- *Lichen sclerosus et atrophius* is an atrophic condition usually seen in postmenopausal women. It differs from leukoplakia in that it is atrophic and does not spread beyond the skin of the vulva itself. Biopsy shows a general thinning of all the layers of the skin; the keratin layer is deficient and the basal papillae are flattened. There is hyaline change in the corium which is infiltrated with lymphocytes.

Psychogenic causes are often invoked where no other cause has been found.

Careful investigation reveals a cause for pruritus vulvae in over 90% of cases. True pruritus must be distinguished from soreness of the vulva, also a common symptom, and often caused by vaginitis, deficiency states and postmenopausal atrophy.

INVESTIGATIONS

This should include:
- a careful *history*, including the use of any substance which might lead to allergy;
- *examination* to determine characteristics and limits of physical signs;
- *bacteriological examination* of vaginal secretions and scrapings from the skin;
- a full *blood count*;
- a *glucose tolerance test* if relevant;
- *biopsy* of the skin of the vulva.

TREATMENT

Women tend to be very sensitive and shy about pruritus and often delay in seeking advice. Self-medication often makes the condition worse.

No treatment should be attempted without full examination and investigation. Blind treatment may mean that a serious condition, such as an early carcinoma or diabetes is overlooked. With full investigation, the cause can be found in almost every case. The help of a dermatologist may be sought in difficult cases. The treatment is that of the cause, e.g., diabetes or anaemia.

Fungus infections should be treated with fungicides such as mycostatin or clotrimazole.

Leukoplakia and lichen sclerosis may respond to ointments or creams containing hydrocortisone. In cases which do not improve, simple vulvectomy may be undertaken.

Care should be taken in using local analgesics, especially benzocaine and amethocaine as acute sensitivity may develop.

LUMP IN THE VULVA

Many conditions may bring a woman complaining of a lump in the vulva.

Conditions of the vulva

- *Congenital.* Hypertrophy of the clitoris or labia minor. If severe, causing discomfort, plastic surgery may be required.
- *Vascular.* Varicose veins of the vulva are often accentuated during pregnancy. If they persist after delivery, they may be treated surgically.
- *Cysts* may occur in the clitoris and the hymen. Sebaceous cysts are common in the skin of the vulva; they may be multiple and some become infected.
- *Infections, boils and carbuncles* may affect the vulva, especially in women with glycosuria and diabetes.
- *Trauma.* Injury to the vulva may lead to a haematoma which can also occur in the puerperium due to secondary haemorrhage.
- *Condylomata.* Three types occur.
  (a) *Condylomata acuminata* (viral warts) are usually multiple, affecting the vulva and the anal region. They present as pedunculated or sessile, branched tumours, growing in clusters like a cauliflower. Small condylomata are treated by podophyllin resin, 0.5%. Large condylomata are best treated surgically by excision with electrical diathermy under general anaesthesia.
  (b) *Condylomata lata* are purplish-grey, flat-topped warty tumours and are a manifestation of secondary syphilis.
  (c) *Molluscum contagiosum* are multiple umbilicate warts on the vulva. Treat as for condylomata acuminata.
- *Swellings of Bartholin's gland.* Cysts of Bartholin's duct and a Bartholin's

abscess are common. Both present as swellings in the fourchette; an acute abscess is painful and tender like a boil. An abscess may rupture spontaneously, but tends to recur. Treatment of both cysts and abscesses is by marsupialization which permits adequate drainage and in many cases the function of the gland is retained. The pus in an abscess should always be cultured and a search made for gonococci in the urethra and cervix, since some Bartholin abscesses are due to gonorrhoea.

• Other benign tumours include the fibroma, lipoma, papilloma and endometrioma.

VAGINAL AND UTERINE CAUSES

A patient complaining of a lump in the vulva may be suffering from:

• prolapse;
• a large polyp;
• inversion of the uterus;
• a vaginal cyst.

INGUINAL CAUSES

A swelling in the inguinal region may present in the labia major and so in the vulva. Causes include:

• inguinal hernia;
• tumour;
• varicocoele of the round ligament;
• hydrocoele of the canal of Nuck.

CONDITIONS OF THE URETHRA

Urethral caruncle occurs mostly in postmenopausal women. It presents as a bright red, exquisitely tender swelling at the posterior margin of the urethral meatus. Symptoms include dysuria, bleeding and dyspareunia. Treatment is to excise the caruncle with diathermy.

Prolapse of the urethra which may be acute or chronic, involves the whole circumference of the urethra and not just the posterior margin of the meatus. It may give similar symptoms to a caruncle. If symptoms are severe, the prolapsed urethra must be excised and repaired.

Carcinoma of the urethra is rare. It may present with dysuria, pain, bleeding or even acute retention of urine. Treatment consists of local radiotherapy with removal of the inguinal lymph glands. If the growth is extensive, the woman may need extensive surgery involving transplantation of the ureters and excision of the bladder and urethra.

MALIGNANT DISEASE OF THE VULVA

Squamous epithelioma

Vulval carcinoma is less common than other gynaecological cancers. The squamous form is the commonest malignant tumour of the vulva. It occurs mainly in the older age group, with a peak incidence at about 60 years of age.

PATHOLOGY

The primary growth is an ulcer with a raised, everted edge and indurated base. Multiple primaries may be found, sometimes the inner side of both labia minora are involved. The growth may also arise on the clitoris.

METHODS OF SPREAD

• The growth may spread by direct extension and contact to other parts of the vulva, vagina or anus.

Secondary spread is mainly by lymphatics. Owing to the rich lymphatic drainage of the vulva, the glands which tend to be involved are:
• superficial inguinal group of both sides;
• inguinal;
• femoral;
• iliac;
• aortic.

In untreated cases, the glands in the groin may break down to form a fungating ulcerated mass of growth.

CLINICAL FEATURES

Carcinoma of the vulva commonly begins as a small nodule, often unnoticed by the patient at first. It grows in size and becomes ulcerated with discharge and bleeding. It tends to grow on the inner surface of the labia minor in elderly women and may remain unnoticed except for slight discomfort and soreness from the discharge until an advanced stage.

DIFFERENTIAL DIAGNOSIS

To differentiate malignancy from other causes of a lump in the vulva or of ulceration is the main problem. All lumps or ulcers of the vulva must be fully investigated including a biopsy.

TREATMENT

Treatment of carcinoma of the vulva is radical vulvectomy, including dissection of all the superficial and deep inguinal glands and possibly the iliac glands. The vulva itself is widely excised in continuity with the mass of tissue containing the glands. Every effort is made to cover the large raw area with skin. Healing may be expedited by the use of skin grafts in some cases (Fig. 4.1). More recently, some surgeons are going back to an incision over each groin and one in the midline other than an *en bloc* dissection. Wide excision in advanced growths may have to include removal of the lower part of the urethra, vagina or anal canal depending on site.

In operable cases, a 5-year cure rate of about 70% is achieved. The prognosis depends mainly on involvement of the lymphatic glands.

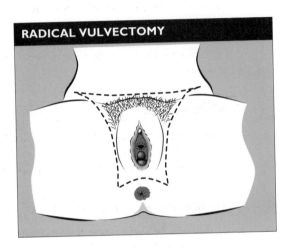

RADICAL VULVECTOMY

Fig. 4.1 The area excised at a radical vulvectomy.

Radiotherapy

Carcinoma of the vulva is relatively radio-resistant while the surrounding normal tissues are radio-sensitive. Hence, it is not employed usually, but high-voltage treatment may be used for recurrences.

Chemotherapy

This is not a primary treatment for squamous epithelioma or cancer of the vulva, but as with carcinomas of the anus it is being used more readily for recurrence.

Adeno-acanthoma

Occasionally seen at the vulva; it is probably a squamous cell metaplasia of an adenocarcinoma. It is of low malignancy and may be treated by wide local excision.

Intra-epithelial carcinoma

In vulval intra-epithelial neoplasia (VIN), the malignant cells are limited to the outer layers of the epidermis and there is no spread to the underlying tissues and no metastases. The whole layer is infiltrated with malignant cells.

CLINICAL FEATURES

The patient has irritation or soreness of the vulva. The appearance may be that of leukoplakia or there may be a red area with a serpiginous outline. VIN may remain dormant for years or may assume the characteristic of invasive carcinoma.

Diagnosis depends on biopsy.

Treatment is by a wide excision with a margin of healthy skin and epithelium.

Basal cell carcinoma

This uncommon tumour presents as an indolent ulcer without invasion of the underlying tissues. Diagnosis is made by biopsy.

The treatment consists of local excision with a margin of normal skin.

Malignant melanoma

Fortunately this highly malignant tumour is rare. It may present as a melanotic nodule or as a pedunculated tumour. The best treatment is to perform radical vulvectomy without previous biopsy. Cases with diffuse spread of melanoma may be treated by radiotherapy.

THE VAGINA

The vagina is lined by stratified squamous epithelium, continuous with that of the vulva below and the ectocervix above, all of which are responsive to oestrogen fluctuation. It shares many pathological problems with these. The major problems are associated with infections which also are common to the vulva and so grouped here.

Infections of the lower genital tract

Natural protection is provided by:
- squamous epithelium thickened by oestrogens;
- low pH(4) by lactic acid derived from intra-epithelial glycogen breakdown;

- mucus from the cervix, Bartholin's gland and Skene's glands rich in bactericidal lysozymes.
   This protection is diminished by a number of causes.
- Pre-pubertal and postmenopausal low oestrogen levels resulting in a thinner epithelium, a higher pH and less mucus production.
- Antibiotics which destroy the normal commensal flora or Doderlein's bacilli.
- Chemical douches which wash away the natural protective secretions.
- Foreign bodies in the vagina such as pessaries or tampons.
- Abortion and menstruation which renders the pH more alkali and removes the protective discharge in the cervical cavity.
- Debilitation.

SYMPTOMS

Vaginal discharge
- Details of the onset, e.g., post coital, post antibiotics.
- The volume—does it soil the clothing or require sanitary towels to be used?
- The colour and consistency:
   (a) white and thick—monilia;
   (b) yellow, green and frothy—trichomonas vaginalis;
   (c) mucus—cervical origin.
   Itchiness or pruritus is commonly associated with monilia and trichomonas.
   Soreness comes with secondary bacterial invasion.
   Ulceration is associated with viral infections or exposure to chemicals, e.g. detergent which causes inflammation.
   An *offensive discharge* is often associated with anaerobic bacterial activity caused by foreign bodies and carcinoma.

EXAMINATION

Inspect the vulva for:
- reddening;
- oedema;
- excoriation from scratching;
- ulceration.
   Inspect the external urethral meatus for prolapse or caruncle.
   Vaginal examination to check for:
- patchy reddening associated with trichomonas;
- white plaques associated with monilia;
- punctate vesicle type ulceration associated with herpes simplex.

Examine the cervix for:

- reddening;
- excessive mucus production;
- tenderness.

Palpate the urethra for thickening and tenderness. Check the Bartholin's glands are not enlarged or tender.

INVESTIGATIONS

Swabs should be taken from the cervical canal, lower urethra, posterior fornix and from any overt lesions on the walls of the lower genital tract. Instant microscopy in saline can sometimes demonstrate the presence of trichomonas and monilia. All the swabs should be sent in Stuart's medium and despatched to the laboratory as soon as possible for culture.

INVESTIGATION OF PARTNER

If the patient is sexually active, then the male partner should have a penile examination with swabs taken from the urethra and the glans.

TREATMENT

The principles of therapy for infection are:

- to avoid indiscriminate treatment;
- to ensure that there is no sexually transmitted disease or carcinoma present;
- to avoid excessive treatment, which may lead to a chemical vaginitis.

MICROBIOLOGY

Gardnerella

This organism is an anaerobe often found as a commensal of the vagina. It is associated with other sexually spread infections.

SYMPTOMS AND SIGNS

There is a vaginal discharge, not dissimilar to that of trichomonas, with a most offensive smell. Occasionally it is the smell alone that brings the patient to the doctor. It is fish-like and is commonly observed more after sexual intercourse. In more severe cases, there will be itching and dyspareunia.

INVESTIGATIONS

A smear may miss the organisms which grow well in a carbon dioxide atmosphere or on blood agar plates. Clue cells on the smear are diagnostic; they are vaginal epithelial cells which appear to have stippled cytoplasma, because each cell is covered with grain positive coccobacteria.

TREATMENT

- Metronidazole 200 mg three times a day for seven days

or

- Tinimidazole 2 g on one occasion.

Such a high proportion of male partners are infected with this organism that it is worth offering treatment automatically as in trichomonas.

Trichomonas

This protozoan organism (Fig. 4.2) readily infects the vagina, often producing severe symptoms, but is usually asymptomatic when it is found in the male colonizing the prepuce, urethra and prostate. It passes between partners at sexual intercourse so both should always be treated.

SYMPTOMS AND SIGNS

The woman has an intensely irritating vaginal discharge with inflammation of the vulva, vagina and cervix. The discharge is often frothy and offensive.

INVESTIGATIONS

A drop of the fresh vaginal smear diluted with saline on which a coverslip is floated allows rapid microscopic diagnosis in the clinic. The motile

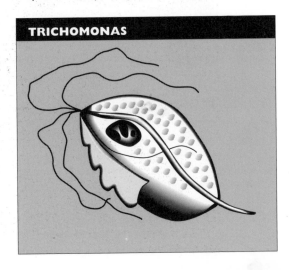

Fig. 4.2 Trichomonas.

organisms swarm all over the slide like dodgem cars. The organism can be cultured.

TREATMENT
- Always treat the partner.
- Metronidazole—200 mg three times a day for seven days

or

- Nimovazole 2 mg—give once after a meal.

Monilia (thrush)

This is caused by a yeast-like fungus (Fig. 4.3). It forms mycelia, but in adverse conditions may become a spore which is resistant to therapy. It thrives in sugar medium and is, therefore, commonly found:
- in pregnancy;
- in diabetes mellitus;
- in oral contraceptive or oestrogen therapy;
- following broad spectrum antibiotics such as tetracycline which kill off the competitive commensal organisms.

SYMPTOMS
- Pruritus vulvae.
- A thick white curd-like discharge.

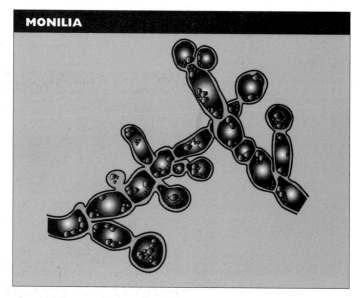

MONILIA

Fig. 4.3 Monilia.

- May be asymptomatic and found incidentally on speculum examination or cervical cytology.

TREATMENT

Local fungicidal pessaries:
- coltrimazole (Canesten) 100 mg for five nights, 200 mg for three nights or 500 mg for one night;
- amphotericin (Fungilin) for three nights;
- miconazole (Gyno-Daktarin) twice a day for 14 days.

Recurrent infections may require systemic therapy:
- ketoconazole (Nizoral) 400 mg with meals for five days;
- itraconazole (Sporanox) 100 mg on two occasions for one day;
- fluconazole (Diflucan) 150 mg once a day;
- the partner should be treated with a corresponding fungicidal cream for local application.

Septic shock syndrome

Caused by a *staphylococcus aureus* septicaemia toxaemia. Associated with:
- obstructed drainage of menses by tampons;
- abrasion of the cervical surface by tampons;
- retrograde flow of menses into the peritoneal cavity.

SYMPTOMS

Shivering, diarrhoea, erythematous rash and fainting. Occurs mostly on second and third days at the peak of menstrual flow.

PHYSICAL SIGNS

- Hypotension.
- Fever.
- Tenderness of vagina and cervix.

TREATMENT

- Removal of tampon.
- Intravenous fluid resuscitation.
- Systemic antibiotics, e.g. Magnapen.

Atrophic vaginitis

Secondary to a lack of oestrogens postmenopausally. The epithelium becomes thin, smooth and shiny with sub-epithelial haemorrhages. Low grade infection from pathogens, which can more easily penetrate the surface, may occur.

SYMPTOMS

- Vulval soreness.
- Superficial dyspareunia.
- Pink discharge.
- Introital shrinking.

PHYSICAL SIGNS

Red shiny epithelium with skin cracking and sub-cuticular haemorrhages. Occasionally causes postmenopausal bleeding. It is important to exclude other causes such as carcinoma.

TREATMENT

If there is secondary infection, antibiotics to which the organism is sensitive may be given. Topical oestrogen creams or pessaries can be used, e.g., dienoestrol or Premarin once or twice a week. This is enough to thicken the epithelium and reduce the pH, but insufficient to produce excessive endometrial stimulation or other causes of bleeding.

FOREIGN BODIES IN VAGINA

This usually presents with a foul discharge caused by the anaerobic organism. This is commonest in:
- children—beads or toys, etc;
- mentally subnormal—beads or coins etc;
- those in custody—vagina used to hide objects (e.g., bank notes), which have been forgotten.

Treatment requires the removal of foreign bodies. Lactic acid pessaries restore pH and encourage regrowth of Doderlein bacilli.

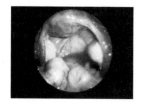

The cervix

Cervicitis, 71
  Acute cervicitis, 71
  Chronic cervicitis, 71
  Cervical erosion of
    ectropion, 71

Cervical polyp, 73
Cancer of the cervix, 73
Cervical interepithelial
  neoplasia (CIN), 75

Treatment of CIN, 76
Treatment of invasive
  carcinoma, 76

The cervix is a hollow muscular cylinder joining the vagina to the uterus. Through it spermatozoa pass upwards for normal conception. In pregnancy, it must help to hold the fetus in the uterus and yet must dilate at childbirth to allow the fetus and placenta to be expelled downwards.

CERVICITIS

Cervicitis may be acute or chronic.

Acute cervicitis

This occurs in acute gonorrhoea and in puerperal and other acute infections of the genital tract (see Chapter 11).

Chronic cervicitis

Chronic infection may follow acute attacks but it usually presents as a part of the syndrome of pelvic inflammatory disease.

Cervical erosion of ectropion

CERVICAL EROSION

The squamous epithelium is missing from the ecto-cervix around the external os. It is replaced by columnar epithelium and patchy areas of granulation tissue which is not as stable and so frequently bleeds and breaks down, being replaced by more heaped up columnar epithelium. Hence, it is not so much an erosion as a piling up or ectropion. There may be mucus secreting glands in an ectropion. The mucus in these may be dammed back producing small mucocoeles.

CONGENITAL EROSION

Columnar epithelium grows down onto the vaginal portion of the cervix in a nulliparous woman as a clearly defined red area surrounding the external os. It is usually symptomless but may produce an increase in mucus secretion. If this becomes infected following coitus, the discharge may become muco-purulent.

ACQUIRED CERVICAL EROSION

This comes most often after childbirth but in most cases heals in a few months. The cervix may be split during delivery and the erosion can then be seen as a red area on each lip. A mucous polyp of the cervix can be associated with cervical erosion and chronic cervicitis.

Women taking combined oral contraceptives may develop a cervical erosion, possibly from the oestrogen causing proliferation of the columnar epithelium.

SYMPTOMS

- *Vaginal discharge* is common and is mucoid except in infected erosions when it becomes mucopurulent.
- *Bloodstained discharge, intermenstrual* or *post coital bleeding* may occur but one should always exclude malignancy.
- *Irritation* or *soreness of the vulva* from the discharge.
- *Micturition symptoms* may include frequency, dysuria or recurrent cystitis; due to trigonitis — remember the close lymphatic connection between the cervix and bladder.
- *Pain* — low sacral backache, deep dyspareunia, and iliac fossa pain.
- *Infertility* can result if the cervical secretions become impermeable to spermatozoa (see Chapter 16). However, cervical erosions are often seen in women attending antenatal clinics.
- *Cervical erosion* may be totally symptomless.

DIAGNOSIS

The diagnosis is made by inspection of the cervix with a speculum. A typical erosion presents as a raised red circular area. It is not friable but may bleed on rubbing. A cervical smear should be taken before any treatment is attempted although if it looks normal, one need not wait for the result before starting therapy.

TREATMENT

A cervical erosion which is found incidentally and causing no symptoms does not require treatment. Those with symptoms of discharge may be treated by:
- Superficial cold cauterization — out-patient procedure.

- Cryocautery—a probe is introduced into the cervix which is frozen to about −50°C for 2 minutes—out-patient procedure.
- Laser cauterization—out-patient procedure.
- Deeper cautery requires an anaesthetic and may be done at the time of other surgery, such as dilatation and curettage (D&C).

After cauterization the patient should be warned to expect some bleeding and a watery discharge. She should also be warned against intercourse for 10 days or so.

CERVICAL POLYP

A cervical polyp is a very common mass seen presenting from the cervix, usually arising in the canal and in most cases benign. It presents a soft bright red tumour of varying size—some may even reach the vulva. It may cause discharge, occasionally bloodstained, and post coital bleeding.

The management is not removing the polyp in the out-patient department. This may be the guardian polyp with other polypi unseen higher up the canal. The woman should be offered a formal hysteroscopy and D&C to exclude other lesions.

All polypi should be submitted to histology. Most will be found to consist of mucus-secreting glands with a supporting stroma, although a few have malignancy changes.

CANCER OF THE CERVIX

Cancer of the cervix arises most frequently from the squamous epithelium at its junction with the columnar epithelium; it is predominantly a squamous carcinoma. A columnar cell type arises from the cervical glands inside the cervical canal, an adenocarcinoma. Malignant change may also arise in a cervical mucous polyp.

AETIOLOGY

- Mainly in the age group 45 to 55.
- Rare in virgins.
- Coitus increases the risk:
  (a) very early coitus;
  (b) multiple sexual partners.
- Infection with the wart virus Types 16 and 18 and certain herpes.
- Common in Negresses but rare in Jewesses or Arab women.
- More frequent in the lower social class groups; possibly hygienic factors may play a part.

PATHOLOGY

95% of the growths are squamous cell carcinomata from the squamo-columnar junction. About 5% are adenocarcinoma from the columnar cells inside the cervical canal.

Invasive cancers present as an ulceration or heaping up of the vaginal portion of the cervix. In advanced cases, the cervix is replaced by an ulcerated, fungated mass of growth which is fixed to the surrounding structures. Spread may be to many areas.

- The vaginal fornices.
- The bladder.
- The body of the uterus.
- The broad ligaments which may cause obstruction of the lower ends of the ureters. A large blood vessel may be eroded with severe haemorrhage.
- Lymphatic spread to the iliac, obturator, sacral, inguinal and para-aortic nodes.
- Blood-stream spread occurs comparatively late but may lead to metastases in the lungs, bones or elsewhere.

SYMPTOMS

The symptoms of cancer of the cervix only begin when the surface of the growth becomes ulcerated. Hence, they appear later with endocervical growths. The chief symptom is a watery *discharge*, often offensive and bloodstained discharge. This is increased by contact after coitus, douching or insertion of a diaphragm. Later frank, sometimes severe and continuous *bleeding* occurs, with the patient rapidly becoming anaemic.

URINARY FREQUENCY

Pain is late, but once it begins it is severe and intractable, radiating from the pelvis and lower back into the legs. Severe nerve root pain follows secondaries in the lumbar vertebrae. *Malaise* and *cachexia* may occur, but loss of weight is not so common.

PHYSICAL SIGNS

Early, the cervix feels hard and bleeds on touch. Later the cervix is ulcerated and friable. In very advanced cases the vaginal vault is filled with an ulcerated mass and pieces of growth are detached by the examining finger; examination may provoke severe bleeding. In endocervical growths the cervix feels barrel-shaped.

The cervical smear may contain frankly malignant cells, but not always because the surface cells are often dead and atypical.

DIAGNOSIS

This depends on biopsy of the cervix which should be combined with curettage of the uterine cavity and the endocervical canal. If the site and size of the lesion allows, a cone biopsy should be taken to include all the squamous-columnar junction and most of the cervical canal.

ANCILLARY METHODS OF DIAGNOSIS

- Colposcopy where the magnified image of the cervix is minutely inspected.
- Schiller's test—painting the cervix with iodine solution. Normal cervix which contains glycogen stains brown but abnormal areas do not stain. It is of major value in indicating those parts of the cervix which should be submitted to biopsy but is not in itself diagnostic.

DIFFERENTIAL DIAGNOSIS

Mainly from:

- cervical erosion or ectropion;
- tuberculosis may present in a proliferative form;
- other chronic granulomatous infections.

STAGING OF CANCER OF THE CERVIX

Stage 0	Intra-epithelial carcinoma (carcinoma in situ). The growth remains within the epithelial layer of the cervix
Stage 1	Cancer clinically limited to the substance of the cervix
Stage 2	Growth has spread to the upper two-thirds of the vagina or into the parametrium but not as far as the pelvic wall
Stage 3	The growth has spread to the lower one-third of the vagina or into the parametrium as far as the lateral pelvic wall
Stage 4	Metastases have formed beyond the pelvis or growth has involved the bladder or the rectum

Box 5.1 Staging of cancer of the cervix.

It must be emphasized that this is a clinical classification; in fact 20% of stage I cases are found at subsequent operation to have metastases in the lymph glands.

CERVICAL INTEREPITHELIAL NEOPLASIA (CIN)

The pre-invasive stage is characterized by dysplasia, the cells lining up in columns. Later there is disorderly arrangement of cells throughout the epithelial layer, and irregular mitoses in the nuclei of the epithelial cells. There are no symptoms and often no abnormal physical signs, the cervix looking normal. CIN may remain non-invasive for years and sometimes probably regresses.

It is generally found in women who are sexually active and is very rare in virgins. The early invasive stage may be characterized by micro-invasion and small numbers of malignant cells are seen invading the deeper layers. There is probably a link between pelvic infection by herpes, human papilloma virus and CIN.

Treatment of CIN

Most cases are diagnosed when a cervical smear contains suspicious or frankly malignant cells. Ideally all such cases should have a colposcopy which permits identification of abnormal epithelium. Biopsy is performed of either the suspicious area or a whole cone is removed of the cervical canal and ectocervix on either side of the squamo-columnar junction. The cone should have its edges through colposcopically normal tissue.

In cases where it seems likely on histological serial examinations that all the abnormal tissue has been excised in the cone biopsy, no further active treatment is required but the patient should be followed up by regular cervical smears. Further pregnancies can be permitted.

An alternative to cone biopsy is the excision of suspicious areas using laser under colposcopic control which allows fine control of the tissue destruction.

Total hysterectomy with conservation of the ovaries may be performed in women who do not want more children and in those who have other symptoms such as menorrhagia. In suitable cases vaginal hysterectomy may be done; a cuff of the vaginal vault must be removed with the uterus whichever route is chosen.

Treatment of invasive carcinoma

The choice of treatment depends on many factors.
- The age and general condition of the patient.
- The extent and type of the lesion.
- Ideally all patients with cancer of the cervix should be seen in consultation by a team of a gynaecologist, a radiotherapist and an oncologist for consideration of all the factors of the individual case.
- The experience, resources and personal preference of the oncology team.

Renal function should be assessed by blood urea and intravenous urography. Urinary infection is often present and should be treated. Anaemia may also need treatment.

Ultrasound or CT scan may help identify spread in the pelvis or to lymph nodes.

Examination under anaesthesia is essential.

- The clinical extent of the growth is assessed.
- Curettage is performed and a biopsy taken in all cases, even those which seem the most obvious clinically.
- A rectal examination is important to exclude invasion of the rectum itself. The clinical extent of growth in the parametrium is also more easily felt rectally.
- Cystoscopy excludes involvement of the bladder.

RADIOTHERAPY

This is the first line of attack in most cases and the treatment of choice with advanced growths or in poor-risk patients. It cannot be used if the bladder is invaded owing to the risk of fistula formation.

Caesium is applied by various techniques; the most common is the Stockholm technique or one of its modifications. A tube containing 50 mg of caesium is put into the uterus and two ovoids or flat boxes containing a further 60 mg are packed into the vagina. Care is taken to give a minimal dose of radiation to the rectum. The caesium is left for 22 hours and three applications are usually given, the second a week after the first and the third two weeks after the second.

An alternative is the use of the cathetron; an empty container is inserted and clamped into position. Several high-intensity cobalt sources are loaded and deliver the irradiation. The apparatus is contained in a sealed unit and radiation delivered by remote control, thus eliminating danger to staff.

Caesium may be used as a preliminary to surgery or combined with external X-ray therapy to the lateral pelvic walls. Advanced techniques of irradiation such as cobalt or the linear accelerator may be used in advanced disease to give total pelvic irradiation.

SURGERY

Surgical excision is suitable for all Stage 1 and many Stage 2 cases. Many surgeons believe that the best results are obtained if preliminary treatment with radiation therapy is followed by a Wertheim's radical abdominal hysterectomy; removing the uterus, tubes, ovaries, broad ligaments and parametrium, the upper half or two-thirds of the vagina and the regional lymph glands (Fig. 5.1).

The Schauta operation is a similar procedure performed by the vaginal route and practised in Europe but rarely in Britain.

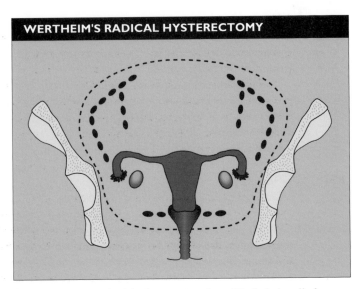

Fig. 5.1 The extent of pelvic tissue removed at a Wertheim's radical abdominal hysterectomy.

PELVIC EXENTERATION

In some advanced cases where carcinoma of the cervix has spread, extensive surgery must be undertaken as the only hope of cure for the patient. It is reserved mainly for patients in good general health with extensive disease involving the bladder or rectum.

Anterior exenteration consists of removing the uterus and adnexae, the vagina, the bladder and the urethra. The ureters are implanted into the colon or into an ileal loop opening on to the abdominal wall.

Posterior exenteration removes the uterus and adnexae, the vagina, descending colon and rectum, leaving a colostomy. This is suitable for posterior growths involving the colon or rectum.

In *total exenteration* the two operations are combined and the patient left with an ileal loop and a colostomy.

RESULTS OF TREATMENT

These are best assessed by a 5-year follow-up and this shows in most centres a cure rate of 70 to 80% with stage I and less than 10% with stage 4.

This range of cure emphasizes the value of early diagnosis and treatment; the tragedy is that so many women do not receive treatment until the disease is advanced.

COMPLICATIONS OF TREATMENT

Complications may follow treatment with irradiation or surgery. Radiotherapy treatment can flair up infection in the renal tract, or exacerbate pelvic abscess. Caesium proctitis may prove troublesome.

The mortality risk at the operation of Wertheim's hysterectomy is now only 1% in experienced hands. In addition to any complications of a severe abdominal operation, there is a risk of ureteric fistula which has been found in about 8% of patients submitted to Wertheim's hysterectomy after irradiation.

PALLIATION

When nothing can be done to cure the patient of cancer, everything concentrates on making her last weeks or months as comfortable as possible. Death may occur mercifully from uraemia or haemorrhage but many women suffer severe and intractable pain in the final stages of the disease.

Analgesics must be used liberally in sufficient amounts to relieve pain. Intrathecal injection of absolute alcohol below the level of the first lumbar vertebra may relieve pain for some months, although with a slight risk of bladder or rectal incontinence. Chordotomy is sometimes used in intractable pain. If there is severe rectal pain, colostomy may be necessary. Morphia and heroin are of great help here and must be retained in the profession's therapeutic armamentarium, prescribing and dispensing being under strict control. Addiction is not a concern in those with advanced pelvic cancer and dosage should be liberal once started.

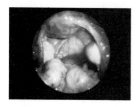

The body of the uterus

Congenital abnormalities, 81

Infections, 82
  Endometritis, 82
  Pyometra, 82
Endometrial polypi, 83

Benign tumours, 83
  Uterine fibroids, 83
  Uterine adenomyosis, 87
Malignant tumours, 88
  Endometrial carcinoma, 88

Rarer tumours, 90
  Sarcoma, 90
  Mixed mesodermal tumours, 90
Chorioncarcinoma, 91

CONGENITAL ABNORMALITIES

Most congenital abnormalities of the uterus relate to either a fusion or a development of Mullerian ducts. The embryology of this is considered in Chapter 2 (Fig. 6.1).

The rarest abnormality is when there is complete failure of fusion leading to a double uterus, a double cervix and two vaginas separated by a septum.

The commonest found abnormalities are a septate vagina alone, a subseptate uterus or a unicornate uterus. Often they are not recognized because they produce no problems.

• *Intercourse* takes place normally in one vagina, pushing the septum to one side.

• *Fertility* and childbearing occurs in a subseptate uterus or a unicornate uterus and often it is not recognized unless a Caesarean section is performed.

• *Pregnancy* in the rudimentary horn of a unicornate uterus could lead to *rupture of the uterus*, but this is most unusual as pregnancies are usually in the dominant horn. Other problems in pregnancy are *pre term labour* or *poor uterine contractions*.

TREATMENT

A vaginal septum is rarely a barrier to delivery, but it is best divided between two artery forceps in the second stage as the head is coming down. Other uterine abnormalities may be treated by unification of the uterus by utriculoplasty (Strassman operation).

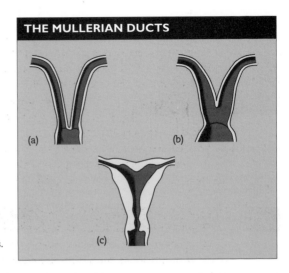

THE MULLERIAN DUCTS

(a)   (b)

(c)

Fig. 6.1 Development of the female genital tract from two Mullerian tubes. (See Fig. 2.22 for details.)

INFECTIONS

Endometritis

The condition is usually acute and associated with ascending infection and may be secondary to cervical infection. The disease may result from:
- post abortal infection;
- criminal abortion;
- excessive curettage;
- intrauterine device infection.

   It rarely results from blood-borne tuberculosis.

FINDINGS

Acute infection
- irregular bleeding;
- uterine tenderness.

Chronic infection
- occasionally secondary amenorrhoea and secondary infertility, caused by the development of intrauterine adhesions leading to partial or complete occlusion of the uterine cavity (Asherman's syndrome).

Pyometra

- Infection leading to pus formation may be associated with blocking of the fallopian tubes and the cervix.

- Pyometra are commoner in older women.
- A bag of pus builds up pressure and distends the uterus causing:
  (a) pain from the stretch of the muscle wall;
  (b) occasional acute bursts of toxaemia as a bolus of pus is forced into a vein and so to the vascular network;
  (c) chronic infection with low grade temperature and malaise;
  (d) occasionally pus is forced through the cervix to produce a purulent or bloodstained discharge.
- Many pyometra are associated with cancer of the endometrium.

Any woman with such symptoms should have a D&C under appropriate antibiotic cover to exclude endometrial malignancy.

ENDOMETRIAL POLYPI

If the endometrium hypertrophies under oestrogen stimulation, areas of it may protrude above the surface producing a sessile or eventually a pedunculated polyp. This may not be shed at the time of menstruation, but form a site for persistent symptoms and signs.

SYMPTOMS

There may be intermenstrual spotting or postmenstrual staining.

SIGNS

There would be no signs, but a hysteroscopy would easily show the polyp.

MANAGEMENT

Endometrial polypi should be removed. Those inside the uterus will require an anaesthetic and have to be twisted off with a polypi forceps. Should the endometrial polyp stalk be long and the polyp present at the cervix, it is probably wise not to remove it in the out-patients department, because this could lead to heavy bleeding. A D&C should be performed at the same time to allow removal of any other polypi that are higher up.

BENIGN TUMOURS

Uterine fibroids

Alternatively named myomata or leiomyomata, uterine fibroids are the commonest of all pelvic tumours. They are benign fibromuscular swellings, arising in the muscle wall of the uterus. Fibroids are oestrogen sensitive.

- Grow fast in pregnancy.
- Shrink:
    (a) at the menopause;
    (b) with anti-gonadotrophic hormone therapy.

Fibroids may be single or multiple (occasionally numbering greater than 100) and vary in size from a seedling to a football. They form a pseudocapsule by compressing surrounding uterine muscle, a process helpful to the surgeon at myomectomy.

AETIOLOGY

Cause is unknown:
- rarely found under the age of 30 years;
- commoner in Afro-Caribbean populations;
- commoner in the nulliparous and women with low fertility;
- often a family history.

PATHOLOGY

- *Subserous*—fibroids just beneath the peritoneum on the outer uterine surface (Fig. 6.2). May become elongated on a stalk (pedunculated) with a risk of torsion and may grow into the broad ligament.
- *Interstitial*—the commonest site for fibroids, surrounded by smooth muscle, enlarging the uterine wall and distorting venous drainage.

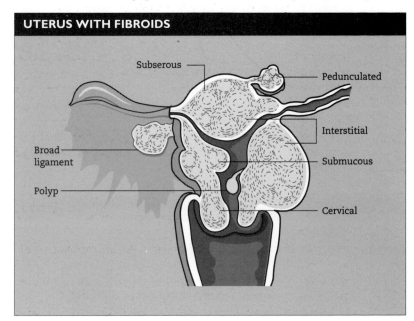

UTERUS WITH FIBROIDS

Subserous — Pedunculated

Interstitial

Broad ligament

Submucous

Polyp

Cervical

Fig. 6.2 Uterus with fibroids.

- *Submucous*—lying immediately below the endometrium and enlarging the surface of the uterine cavity sometimes leading to menorrhagia. Fibroids may become pedunculated forming polypi which can even extrude through the cervix.

DEGENERATION

Uterine fibroids frequently outgrow their blood supply and degenerate.

- *Hyaline*—an aseptic necrosis with loss of muscle cell structure. This may lead to calcification.
- *Cystic*—a sequel to hyaline change with subsequent breakdown and cyst formation giving a honeycomb appearance.
- *Fatty*—in which partial necrosis results in the development of fatty substances which may subsequently undergo calcification (visible on X-rays and ultrasound).
- *Red*—necrobiosis, particularly encountered in the mid trimester of pregnancy or the early puerperium. This breakdown of blood supply by thrombosis leads to necrosis and suffusion with red blood cells.
- *Sarcomatous*—rare malignant change reported in 0.2 to 0.4% of fibroids examined in asymptomatic older women at autopsy.

SYMPTOMS

- *None*—a pelvic swelling is found incidentally on examination.
- Occasional *tightness* of waistband of clothes.
- *Pressure*—bladder compression causing daytime frequency and occasionally impaired urinary stream. In the supporting ligaments it causes backache and overall sensation of pelvic heaviness.
- *Pain*—associated with red degeneration or torsion of subserous pedicles.
- *Menstrual disturbances*:
    (a) menorrhagia—heavy bleeding and prolonged menstruation;
    (b) irregular menses—often associated with submucous fibroids and polypi.

INVESTIGATIONS

- Ultrasound—to define the location, the dimensions and the consistency.
- Laparoscopy—undertaken if clinical and ultrasonic investigations are inconclusive.

DIAGNOSIS

Bimanual palpation reveals hard rounded non-tender often bosselated mass, moving when the cervix is displaced.

DIFFERENTIAL DIAGNOSIS

- Pregnancy—particularly if fibroids have been softened by cystic degeneration.
- Ovarian tumour—often cystic, unilateral and does not move with cervical displacement.
- Adenomyosis—which more commonly causes uniform diffuse and tender uterine enlargement.

TREATMENT

- If small and asymptomatic, conservative management with annual examination and ultrasound monitoring of size is sufficient. This is especially used in women over 40 because fibroids do not grow after menopause and may shrink.
- Menstrual or pressure symptoms rarely may dictate surgery.
- Pain—requires analgesia.
- Heavier and longer periods are the commonest indication for proceeding to surgery.

SURGERY

- Abdominal hysterectomy—suitable when family is complete with women over the age of 40 or when the uterus is grossly enlarged and distorted by multiple fibroids.
- Vaginal hysterectomy—when fibroids are small and few in number and there is an associated prolapse of the uterus.
- Myomectomy—in young women whose families are incomplete or when there is a personal desire to retain the uterus. The procedure is often vascular and may cause scarring, with adhesion formation impairing fertility. If the fibroids are numerous it is impossible to remove them all, and growth of the remainder may cause problems in the future. The technique involves making an incision over the fibroid and shelling it out from the pseudocapsule, then resuturing the raw area, usually in two layers (Fig. 6.3).

EFFECTS ON CHILDBEARING

- Implantation over a fibroid may lead to spontaneous abortion.
- Pain may develop from red degeneration.
- Premature labour may develop if the fibroids are large and multiple.
- Dysfunctional uterine contractions may follow the interruption of smooth waves of electrical stimulation by masses of inert, non-myometrial tissue.
- The pelvis may be obstructed causing malpresentation or even obstructed labour. This is unusual because most fibroids usually move up as the uterus grows in pregnancy, whilst cervical fibroids do not.

MYOMECTOMY

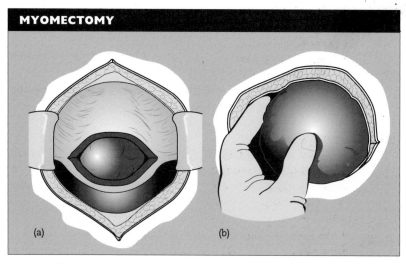

(a)

(b)

Fig. 6.3 A fibroid is shelled out through the pseudocapsule at the myomectomy. (a) The linear curved cut in the uterine muscle and fibroid soon gapes under pressure through to the pseudocapsule. (b) A finger shells out the fibroid from the pseudocapsule.

- Post partum haemorrhage and retained placenta are more common.
- Management in pregnancy is conservative. The aim should be to secure a vaginal delivery. If a Caesarean section becomes necessary, the incision in the uterus should be manoeuvred around the fibroids. They should not be removed or incised as severe haemorrhage may develop leading to the need for a hysterectomy.

UTERINE ADENOMYOSIS

Adenomyosis is a condition where endometrial glands of stroma are found within the uterine musculature. If localized to one site, it is called an adenomyoma. It is like a diffuse endometriosis in the muscle of the uterus.

PATHOLOGY

The uterus is enlarged and thick walled with no pseudocapsule formation, as in fibroids. The endometrial glands often do not menstruate, as they derive from the basal layer of the endometrium.

SYMPTOMS

This condition is most frequent in women aged 35 to 40, with reduced fertility. The symptoms usually are:

- congestive dysmenorrhoea;
- menorrhagia;
- dyspareunia.

SIGNS

A uniformly enlarged uterus which is rarely larger than 12 cm. It is tender on palpation, particularly premenstrually.

DIFFERENTIAL DIAGNOSIS

- Uterine fibroids.
- Early pregnancy.
- Uterine infection.

TREATMENT

- Conservative use of progestational therapy, e.g. norethisterone 10 to 20 mg daily.
- Danazol 200 to 400 mg daily.
- Anti-gonadotrophins: buserelin or goserelin (Chapter 12).

All hormone regimes aim to suppress menstruation, but each carries side effects and usually cannot be used for more than some months at a time.

SURGERY

Abdominal hysterectomy is the treatment of choice, although occasionally resection of the affected area can be considered.

MALIGNANT TUMOURS

Endometrial carcinoma

AETIOLOGY

- Mean age of presentation is 56 years. Four fifths of the women are menopausal and it is rare under the age of 40.
- Associated with hyperoestrogenic states:
  (a) obesity;
  (b) diabetes;
  (c) late menopause;
  (d) prolonged use of unopposed oestrogens;
  (e) oestrogen secreting tumours.
- May be associated with:
  (a) previous pelvic irradiation;
  (b) lower parity.

PATHOLOGY

- Usually an adenocarcinoma.
- More often well differentiated than anaplastic.
- May be associated with squamous metaplasia where, if excessive, becomes an adenocanthoma.
- May be associated with pyometra or haematometra, secondary to cervical stenosis.
- Spreads by invasion through the myometrium and by filling the uterine cavity.
- Invasion to the cervix with subsequent lymphatic spread involving the iliac and para-aortic nodes.
- Tumours of upper uterus may spread along the lymphatics in the round ligaments to the deep inguinal nodes.
- In advanced cases, the blood-stream spread may carry to the lungs, liver and to the bones.

SYMPTOMS

- Postmenopausal bleeding: this symptom should be assumed to be caused by carcinoma of the endometrium until proved otherwise.
- Blood stained discharge.
- Irregular bleeding.

SIGNS

- Less commonly, uterine enlargement.
- Bleeding through the cervix.

INVESTIGATIONS

- Ultrasound to assess dimensions of any tumour and to show endometrial thickness.
- Cytology brush from lower cervical canal and posterior fornix to analyse the cells.
- Hysteroscopy to locate the site of origin of the bleeding, its extent and to ensure an adequate biopsy is taken. Beware perforation as the uterine wall is often friable.

STAGING

Box 6.1 shows the clinical staging of endometrial cancer.

TREATMENT

The treatment of uterine carcinoma is usually surgical.

- If the uterus is small and the tumour well differentiated, a total abdominal hysterectomy and bilateral salpingo-oophorectomy is performed.
- If the uterus is enlarged but the tumour confined to the upper part of

---

CLINICAL STAGING OF ENDOMETRIAL CANCER

Stage 0   Histology suspicious of invasive cancer but inconclusive
Stage 1   Carcinoma confined to the body of the uterus
Stage 2   Extension to the cervix
Stage 3   Extension outside the uterus but within the true pelvis
Stage 4   Involvement of the:
          (a) bladder
          (b) rectum
          (c) extension outside the true pelvis

Box 6.1 Clinical staging of endometrial cancer.

the corpus, an extended hysterectomy with bilateral salpingo-oophorectomy removing a cuff of the vagina is indicated.
• If the cervix shows signs of invasion, a Wertheim's hysterectomy which includes removal of the upper half of the vagina and pelvic lymph nodes is the best surgery.

Radiotherapy is rarely employed alone. It may be used:
• if there is deep invasion of the myometrium;
• if there is evidence of node involvement at surgery.

Hormone therapy—progestogens inhibit the rate of growth and spread of endometrial carcinoma:
• Depo-Provera—100mg prior to surgery and 100mg intra-muscularly each month following surgery.

RARER TUMOURS

Sarcoma

Occurs in:
• childhood as sarcoma botryoides;
• postmenopausal women with a fibroid.

It is highly malignant, radio-resistant, spreads by the blood-stream and diagnosed late. Treatment is a total abdominal hysterectomy and bilateral salpingo-oophorectomy. Recurrences are treated with actinomycin or progestogens.

Mixed mesodermal tumours

These arise from mesodermal cells of the ovarian ducts and may contain primitive muscle cells, myxomatous tissue, cartilage and glands. They present with abnormal bleeding and treatment is by hysterectomy or occasionally by exenteration. Vascular spread is common, prognosis poor.

Chorioncarcinoma

A malignant tumour arising from chorionic tissue following a hydatidiform mole, abortion or pregnancy. It is recognized by tumour marker as they all secrete hCG (Chapter 21).

CHAPTER 7

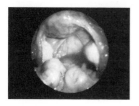

The fallopian tubes

Congenital abnormalities, 93

Torsion of the fallopian tube, 93

Salpingitis, 93

Acute salpingitis, 94

Chronic salpingitis, 95

Tuberculous salpingitis, 96

Pelvic thrombophlebitis, 97

Ectopic pregnancy, 97

Unruptured ectopic, 98

Ruptured ectopic, 99

Benign tumours of the tube, 101

Carcinoma of the tube, 101

CONGENITAL ABNORMALITIES

The fallopian tubes are developed from the Mullerian ducts. Occasionally one or both may be missing, leading to relative or obviously complete infertility.

Accessory ostia on the anti-mesenteric border of the tube are not uncommon and usually have no effect on fertility. These may be surrounded by mini-fimbria.

Reduplication of the fallopian tubes are exceedingly rare, but have been reported.

TORSION OF THE FALLOPIAN TUBE

This rare cause of lower abdominal pain is usually associated with ovarian torsion when the ovary is on a long pedicle. Treatment depends upon the degree of devascularization of the tube and ovary:
- if on unwinding the tissues are healthy, they are best conserved with a securing suture to the side wall of the pelvis to prevent retorsion;
- if the tissues are devitalized, the ovary and tube must be removed.

SALPINGITIS

An ascending infection from the vagina through the cervix is the usual cause of salpingitis. It is often associated with:
- intercourse;
- transcervical surgery (D&C or evacuation);
- intrauterine foreign bodies such as an intrauterine device (IUD);
- retained products of conception;
- very rarely blood-borne infection.

ACUTE SALPINGITIS

The fallopian tubes become red, swollen and distorted, often obstructed at the abdominal end so a pyosalpinx forms. Peritoneal inflammation with adhesions to the serosal surface occurs, leading to pelvic abscess and, if severe, to septicaemia. The condition is usually bilateral. The destruction of the cilia lining of the tube leads to infertility. Chronic hydrosalpinges may become reinfected.

CLINICAL FEATURES
- Pyrexia, often with a temperature higher than 39°C.
- Tachycardia.
- Dehydration.

ABDOMINAL EXAMINATION
- Lower abdominal pain with guarding.
- If parietal peritoneum is involved, rebound tenderness.
- Distension.

VAGINAL EXAMINATION
- Cervical excitation pain.
- Immobilized fixed uterus.
- Fullness in the fornices and tenderness over the tubes.

INVESTIGATIONS
- Organisms may be isolated from cervical discharge.
- *Escherichia coli*, haemolytic streptococcus and staphylococcus are often found in the puerperium and post abortion.
- *Clostridium welchii* may thrive in the presence of dead tissue, e.g., placental products.
- Leucocytosis (in excess of $20 \times 10^9/l$).
- Laparoscopy is the only certain way of making a true diagnosis. Remember to take serosal swabs.

DIFFERENTIAL DIAGNOSIS
- *Appendicitis* — pain is usually central then radiating to the right iliac fossa; the fever is lower.
- *Ruptured ectopic pregnancy* — if there is intra-peritoneal bleeding, symptoms such as faintness and shoulder tip pain. Tenderness tends to be unilateral and a pregnancy test is usually positive.
- *Ovarian tumour torsion* — The pain is localized and unilateral. Pregnancy test is negative and there is no pyrexia. Ultrasound will confirm.
- *Pyelonephritis* — The pain is usually associated with loin tenderness and there are pus cells in the urine.

- *Intestinal obstruction*—usually associated with colicky pain and abdominal distension. X-rays show fluid levels.

TREATMENT

Conservative
- Sit the patient upright in bed.
- Set up intravenous infusion.
- Administer broad spectrum antibiotics until the high vaginal swab (HVS) microbiology and sensitivity reports have been returned.
- Drugs such as Augmentin, cephradine or Flagyl are suitable. Continue the antibiotics after the acute phase for two to three weeks.
- Provide analgesia.

Radical
- Exploratory surgery should be contemplated if diagnosis is in doubt.
- Use only minimal interference, e.g., drainage under antibiotic cover.

CHRONIC SALPINGITIS

Chronic salpingitis is usually a sequel to acute or subacute infections but is often associated with a lower grade purulent organism.

PATHOLOGY
- Thickened fallopian tubes.
- Fibrosis.
- Hydrosalpinges.
- Pelvic floor peritoneal adhesions.

SYMPTOMS
- Present recurrent episodes of low abdominal pain.
- Deep dyspareunia.
- Congestive dysmenorrhoea.
- Heavy periods.
- Infertility.

INVESTIGATIONS
- Ultrasound scan of pelvis.
- Laparoscopy. If there is no recent acute episode, dye installation with antibiotic cover.

LONG TERM SEQUELAE
- Infertility.
- Ectopic pregnancy.

TUBERCULOUS SALPINGITIS

Although this blood-borne infection is rarely encountered in the Western World it is still common in the Third World.

INFECTION

Secondary to pulmonary lesions.

- The infection spreads from the fallopian tube epithelium into the musculature and finally involves the serosal peritoneum where miliary tubercles form.
- Often associated with pyosalpinx, containing caseous pus (occasionally calcified).
- 85% of cases are associated with endometrial involvement as well.

DIAGNOSIS

- Hysteroscopy or diagnostic curettage.
- Histology which may show giant cell epithelioid and round cells.
- Ziehl–Nielsen staining may demonstrate a lesion.
- Guinea pig inoculation grows systemic tuberculosis.

PRESENTATION

- The infection is usually found incidentally at the time of infertility investigations.
- Occasionally associated with amenorrhoea if the endometrium is involved.
- Rarely presents with night fever, sweats, malaise and weight loss.

TREATMENT

Cultured organisms should be submitted to sensitivity tests to:

- streptomycin;
- para-aminosalicyclic acid;
- rifampicin;
- isoniazid with close long-term monitoring.

Long-term follow-up and investigations are essential to ensure that there is not an active focus of tuberculosis elsewhere in the body; therefore chest X-ray and renal scanning are required.

PROGNOSIS

The cure of the disease is associated with excellent results but the tube damage is irreparable.

PELVIC THROMBOPHLEBITIS

Pelvic thrombophlebitis is usually a sequel to severe pelvic infections, especially with an anaerobic streptococcus.

PRESENTATION

- Lower abdominal pain and low grade fever.
- Exacerbations of fever associated with pleuritic pain if pulmonary embolization takes place.
- Occasionally involvement of the common iliac vein and oedema of the legs develops.

ECTOPIC PREGNANCY

An ectopic pregnancy is an extrauterine pregnancy; the commonest site is the fallopian tube. It may also occur, though rarely, in:

- the cervix;
- the uterine cornu;
- the ovary;
- the abdominal cavity and broad ligament.

For practical purposes, ectopic pregnancy will be considered as tubal pregnancy.

INCIDENCE

In the UK, it is about one in every 200 pregnancies. In other countries, especially if there is a large black population, it may be higher.

CAUSES

The ovum is usually fertilized in the fallopian tube and reaches the uterus in about five or six days, but the trophoblast is sufficiently developed for implantation to take place before this. Anything delaying the fertilized ovum will result in tubal pregnancy.

- *Salpingitis* is the commonest predisposing cause. It may not be so severe as to cause complete closure of the tube, but it may destroy the tubal cilia or cause kinking with stricture of the tube.
- *Congenital malformation* may lead to crypts and diverticula.
- *Endometriosis* of the tube narrows it, and the ovum may implant at such sites.
- *Contra-lateral implantation*—the fertilized ovum may come from one ovary but be carried into the opposite tube, so that the passage takes longer and trophoblast develops so much that implantation takes place in the tube. In such cases the tubal pregnancy will be on one side and the corpus luteum of the pregnancy in the opposite ovary.

PATHOLOGY

The embryo cannot grow beyond a certain size in the tube; the trophoblast gradually erodes the tubal wall with its blood vessels and eventually bleeding takes place.

A tubal pregnancy may finish in a number of ways.

- *Absorption*—in a few cases absorption of a very early tubal pregnancy occurs.
- *Tubal mole*—this is a common termination. The embryo dies in the tube with a small amount of bleeding and is retained in the tube in a ball of clot.
- *Pelvic haematocoele*—bleeding is more extensive and a collection of blood forms in the pouch of Douglas. This is often associated with tubal abortion, the products of conception being expelled from the tube into the peritoneal cavity.
- *Tubal rupture*—this is the most dramatic outcome, though less common than tubal mole or tubal abortion. The tube may rupture with acute intraperitoneal haemorrhage from erosion of an artery. The pregnancy is often implanted in the isthmus of the tube.
- *Secondary abdominal pregnancy*—this is the rarest outcome. The embryo is expelled complete from the tube and acquires a secondary attachment in the peritoneal cavity.

Full term abdominal pregnancy is one of the rarities of obstetric practice and delivery must be by laparotomy. Normal children can be delivered from the peritoneal cavity, but others develop gross deformities or die before delivery.

CLINICAL FEATURES

Symptoms of ectopic pregnancy.

- *Amenorrhoea* of early pregnancy. This is not always there if the ectopic presents early.
- *Pain*—cramp-like and colicky at first and often unilateral due to spasm of the tubal muscle.
- *Bleeding*—when a pregnancy implants in the tube, the uterine endometrium is converted into decidua; when parts of it separate there is resultant bleeding. Such bleeding is usually scanty, less than a normal period, and dark brown in colour.

Unruptured ectopic

The physical signs of an undisturbed ectopic pregnancy are:
- possibly slight activity of the breasts;
- on lower abdominal examination, there can be slight tenderness on one side more than the other and at bimanual examination the cervix is

soft and the uterus slightly enlarged; there may be dark blood oozing from the external os;

- the pregnant tube may be felt as a tender ill-defined swelling to one side of the uterus (Fig. 7.1).

A tubal mole gives a similar clinical picture but the mole is generally easily palpable as an only slightly tender swelling in the lateral fornix.

A pelvic haematocoele is a collection of blood in the pouch of Douglas. It can present with abdominal and pelvic pain. An abdominal mass may be palpable. On bimanual examination, the haematocoele is felt as a diffuse boggy swelling. If it is of any size, it displaces the uterus to the opposite side of the pelvis.

DIFFERENTIAL DIAGNOSIS

- Retroverted gravid uterus.
- Torsion or haemorrhage in an ovarian cyst.
- A pyosalpinx.
- A degenerating fibroid.
- Carcinoma of the ovary in an older woman.

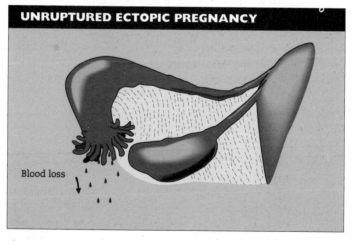

UNRUPTURED ECTOPIC PREGNANCY

Blood loss

Fig. 7.1 Unruptured ectopic pregnancy at the lateral end of the tube.

Ruptured ectopic (Fig. 7.2)

Acute rupture presents as an abdominal acute incident. The woman collapses with severe abdominal pain; if bleeding goes on, she has pallor, shock, rapid pulse, hypotension and air hunger.

The abdomen is slightly distended, tender and rigid. The uterus is rigid and slightly enlarged. Palpation of a tender mass is unlikely because of the guarding.

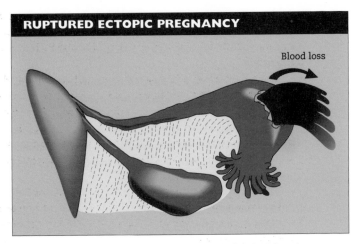

Fig. 7.2 Ruptured ectopic pregnancy at the medial end of the tube.

DIFFERENTIAL DIAGNOSIS

Differentiate from any other abdominal catastrophes such as rupture of a viscus or acute peritonitis. The clinical picture of a ruptured ectopic is so typical that in most cases diagnosis presents no difficulty. Causes to be considered include:

- a haemorrhagic corpus luteum;
- haemorrhage into a small ovarian cyst;
- pelvic appendicitis;
- salpingitis;
- incomplete uterine abortion.

DIAGNOSIS

Diagnosis is usually made on the clinical findings. Investigations include:

- a pregnancy test;
- ultrasound is helpful by excluding an intrauterine pregnancy and the presence of blood in the pouch of Douglas—the tubal mass is often not seen;
- diagnostic laparoscopy with preparations for further surgery if there is blood in the pelvis.

TREATMENT

An intravenous drip should be set up and a blood transfusion given as soon as possible. It is sometimes possible later to collect the extravasated blood from the peritoneal cavity and reinject it. There will be no compatability problems, although the spilt blood may be short of clotting agents.

The treatment of tubal pregnancy used to be a laparotomy with removal of the affected tube. If the tube is not seriously damaged, it may be possible to conserve it, leaving the woman with a chance of conception.

In a case of suspected rupture with severe haemorrhage, the woman must be taken to the operating theatre immediately. Little time should be spent attempting resuscitation; this is time wasted and may only increase bleeding. Using laparoscopy, it is sometimes possible to perform tubal surgery. If not, a laparotomy will be needed to clamp off the bleeding zone of the tube. Alternatively, fetocidal drugs (e.g., methotrexate) can be directly injected.

In most cases, the affected tube should be removed; an exception may be made if the woman desires children or if the other tube is missing or seriously diseased. If a tube is left, there is a distinct risk of recurrence of ectopic pregnancy.

Tubal pregnancy and normal intrauterine pregnancy can very rarely occur at the same time.

BENIGN TUMOURS OF THE TUBE

Cysts may arise in the fimbria which occasionally undergo torsion.

Adenomyoma of smooth muscle and glands can occur in the muscle, pressing into the cavity.

CARCINOMA OF THE TUBE

Primary
• A rare malignancy occurring in older women.
• Papillary carcinoma (not adenocarcinoma) may be solid or alveolar.
• Sometimes there is a vaginal discharge of an orange-yellow colour.
  Treatment is as for ovarian carcinoma.
Secondary
• Metastases in the tube most commonly come from cancer of the ovary or uterus.

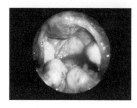

The ovaries

Congenital abnormalities,
103
Infections, 104
Diagnosis, 104
  Features of common
  tumours, 105

Cysts, 105
New growths, 106
Carcinoma of the ovary,
110

Spread of ovarian
  carcinoma, 110
Treatment of ovarian
  tumours, 112

The ovaries are a pair of solid organs suspended behind the broad ligaments in the pelvis. They subserve two functions.
• The production of oocytes from the germinal epithelium during the reproductive years of a woman's life.
• The production of steroid hormones, mostly oestrogen, from the stroma. This function goes on for longer than the reproduction years, but fades in the decade afterwards.

CONGENITAL ABNORMALITIES

The ovaries derive from the germinal ridge at the back of the coelomic cavity, starting to develop high up in the region of the kidneys. They travel down in fetal life drawn by the gubernacula. It is extremely rare for the ovaries to be missing; a most unusual abnormality associated with primary amenorrhoea, but not necessarily with a change of secondary sexual characteristics.

Occasionally, small clumps of ovarian tissue are left on the pelvic course of the migration of the ovary, making *accessory ovarian tissue*. These can function, but are more likely to produce hormones than oocytes.

The commonest group of congenital abnormalities are the various gonadal dysgenesis syndromes such as Turner's syndrome. These are dealt with under functional problems of gynaecology.

The resistant ovary syndrome, where the woman appears to have normal secondary sexual characteristics and primary follicles are present on ovarian biopsy could be considered as a congenital abnormality. The karyotype is normal and the condition is probably due to abnormal gonadotrophin receptors.

INFECTIONS

Pure oophoritis is rare. However, the ovary is often involved in general pelvic infection. The condition of salpingo-parametro-oophoritis is probably a better description of what is usually called chronic salpingitis.

Certain viral conditions such as mumps can affect the ovary, and can cause ovarian swelling and some upset in ovulation, although this is very rare. Unlike such infections in the male, this is usually temporary.

TUMOURS

HISTORY

Enlargement of the ovary often occurs without any symptoms, for the ovaries are tucked away in the pelvis and can expand without causing very much pressure on surrounding organs until they get quite large. Pain is not a usual association nor is vaginal bleeding, except with the few hormone manufacturing ovarian tumours.

SYMPTOMS

When ovarian tumours do produce symptoms they are varied.

• *Abdominal distension* — this is usually noticed by the woman herself with an increase of skirt size or when washing in the bath. Usually the tumour has to be greater than 14 cm in diameter before she notices it and often, in the mildly plump, it could be missed until 20 cm.

• *Pressure* on the rectum, bladder or lymphatic system producing appropriate pressure or damming back symptoms.

• *Pain* — this is usually associated with complications of tumours:
    (a) torsion;
    (b) rupture;
    (c) haemorrhage. (These are dealt with in detail in Chapter 22.)

• *Hormone secretion* — this only happens with a few rare tumours. They may synthesize either:
    (a) oestrogens — leading to menstrual upset (e.g., granuloma cell tumours);
    (b) androgens — leading to masculinization including amenorrhoea (e.g., arrhenoblastoma).

EXAMINATION

The woman may look cachectic and show signs of weight loss if presenting with malignant tumours of the ovary. Otherwise, there are few general signs:

• The *abdomen* may appear enlarged. If there is gross stretch of the abdominal wall, there may be shiny skin with possible oedema and *peau d'orange*.

- *Palpation* may allow a firm ovarian cyst to be felt. If there is ascites or the cyst is lax, it might be difficult to delineate it.
- *Percussion* may demonstrate central dullness with resonance of the flanks. However, if ascites is present, this sign is lost and shifting dullness may replace it.
- *Auscultation* is usually not helpful.
- *Pelvic examination* may reveal a tumour.

Paradoxically, smaller tumours are often easier to feel than the larger ones.

If benign, the mass can be felt separate from the uterine body and may be freely mobile. If it is fixed, infection, endometriosis or malignancy should be suspected.

Some cysts appear to be anterior to the uterus and they should not surprise the student. However, if they arise from the ovary behind the uterus, firmer cysts such as dermoids can extend to the front of the uterus and thus give a confusing picture.

INVESTIGATIONS

Ultrasound of the abdomen can detect masses and ascites; with smaller masses, a vaginal probe approach is even better at delineation. X-rays are not very helpful unless calcification is present (e.g., dermoids).

Some tumour marker blood concentrations are raised, e.g., CA_{125}. However, they are probably of more use in screening tests (see Chapter 17) than confirming a clinical diagnosis which is best done by ultrasound.

Features of common tumours

It is difficult to classify ovarian masses precisely, for the ovary has several histological tissues in it and each can contribute to ovarian tumours. Many are simple variations of normal physiology.

Cysts

FOLLICULAR CYSTS

These consist of unruptured and enlarged Graafian follicles and a normal ovary commonly contains one or more small cysts (less than 5 cm in diameter). They are not neoplastic and tend to disappear by resorption of fluid. These cysts rarely exceed 15 cm in diameter and are lined with one or more layers of granulosa cells which degenerates in longstanding cysts. There may be difficulty clinically in distinguishing a follicular cyst from a small serous cystadenoma.

Multiple follicular cysts are found in:
- metropathia haemorrhagica with cystic hyperplasia of the endometrium;
- polycystic ovary syndrome with stromal hyperplasia of the ovary.

CORPUS LUTEUM CYSTS

These are lined with luteal cells derived from the granulosa layer. The corpus luteum of pregnancy may reach 3 cm or more in diameter and appear cystic. Sometimes, apart from pregnancy, the corpus luteum persists, becoming cystic and causing amenorrhoea followed by bleeding. Haemorrhage into a corpus luteum can cause pain and the symptoms and signs may resemble those of ectopic pregnancy (Chapter 22).

HAEMORRHAGIC CYSTS

A haemorrhagic cyst may result from bleeding into a Graafian follicle or corpus luteum. Sometimes acute symptoms result, leading to laparotomy. Removal of the ovary may be performed unnecessarily in young women. All that is required is haemostasis of the affected area after shelling out the haematoma.

THECA LUTEAL CYSTS

Theca luteal cysts are found in association with raised hCG levels:
- hydatidiform mole;
- chorioncarcinoma;
- gonadotrophin therapy.

Both ovaries are enlarged (10 cm or more) with multiple cysts lined by luteal cells. The ovaries return to normal when hCG levels reduce.

GERMINAL INCLUSION CYSTS

These microscopic cysts are formed by down-growth of the germinal epithelium; microscopic cystic spaces in the ovarian stroma. They have no pathological or clinical significance.

NEW GROWTHS

SEROUS CYSTADENOMA

This benign tumour contains fluid which is rich in protein, resembling blood serum. It often contains papillary growths each with a connective tissue core with a covering of cubical cells, similar to those which line the cyst. In larger cysts, papillae are always present and in some cases grow rapidly, almost filling the cyst and giving the appearance of a solid tumour.

Bilateral tumours are often seen and malignant change is frequent. The histological diagnosis of malignancy is occasionally not easy and may have to be made on the clinical features.

MUCINOUS CYSTADENOMA

This is the commonest of the benign new growths. It contains viscous mucin, the secretion of the lining of the tumour. The cyst grows slowly and may reach a very large size, so as to fill the abdominal cavity. Tumours over 100 kg have been reported (i.e., heavier than the woman from whom they are taken).

It is multilocular, each loculus being lined with a tall columnar epithelium which may be ciliated and can proliferate to form papillary folds. Goblet cells are found among the epithelial cells.

The origin of these tumours is disputed. They may arise from:
• rests of Mullerian epithelium in the ovary;
• rests of hind-gut epithelium, also columnar celled and mucus secreting, carried into the ovary during intrauterine life.

Malignant change occurs in about 5%.

PSEUDOMYXOMA PERITONEI

This is a rare condition whereas mucinous tumours are common; it may occur if the contents of a cyst leak or are spilled into the peritoneal cavity. Epithelial cells lining the cyst proliferate and produce a mucinous ascites, the whole peritoneal cavity becoming filled with viscid mucinous material. The condition arises also from a mucocoele of the appendix and thus may be found in males as well as females.

FIBROADENOMA

This benign tumour occurs in about 3% of women with an ovarian tumour. It arises from connective tissue as a solid non-encapsulated tumour which may be bilateral and can grow to 20 cm. The normal ovary is compressed but not invaded. The histological appearance is that of a benign tumour composed of whorls of fibrous connective tissue resembling the ovarian stroma. These tumours are associated with:
• ascites;
• hydrothorax—only occasionally;
• hydropericardium.

This association is Meigs' syndrome and is also found with a Brenner tumour, granulosa cell or theca cell tumours. The effusions into the serous cavities disappear when the tumour is removed.

BRENNER TUMOUR

This rare tumour is found mostly in postmenopausal women, often discovered accidentally at autopsy since it remains small and symptomless. It is a mostly solid tumour with nests of epithelial cells resembling transitional epithelium enclosed in dense fibrous tissue. Cavities arising in the epithelial nests contain mucin like mucinous cystadenoma. A Brenner tumour is sometimes found in a mucinous cystadenoma. Meigs' syndrome may occur.

MESONEPHROMA

This is an uncommon tumour characterized by glomerular structures and tubules lined by hobnail cells. It may be benign or malignant and is found in all ages. It appears not only in the ovary but in the cervix, vagina and broad ligament, along the line of the mesonephric duct.

GERM CELL TUMOURS

This is a group of primitive germ cell tumours. The best known is the *dysgerminoma*. This rare tumour arises from primitive undifferentiated sex cells; histologically identical tumours are found in the ovary (dysgerminoma) and in the testicle (seminoma). It consists of epithelial cells arranged in alveoli separated by septa of fibrous tissue infiltrated with round cells, resembling lymphocytes. The epithelial cells are large and round or polygonal, like spermatocytes. It may happen in young patients and is liable to malignant change in both sexes. Dysgerminoma is more common in individuals with infantile genitalia and in males with undescended testicles, but it also occurs in normal individuals. It secretes gonadotrophin so that a positive pregnancy test may be obtained.

Endodermal sinus tumour or *embryonal carcinoma* may occur with dysgerminoma.

DERMOID OR BENIGN TERATOMA

This common tumour of the ovary makes up 15% of all ovarian tumours. It occurs mainly between 15 and 30 years and is the commonest tumour in this age group because it develops from an unfertilized ovum by parthenogenesis and thus occurs at the height of the reproductive period. These tumours are often multiple and bilateral.

A dermoid is a thick walled cyst with solid parts, rarely exceeding 20 cm in diameter. It does not adhere to surrounding structures so torsion is common. The cyst is lined by squamous epithelium and contains:

- a fatty pultaceous secretion resembling sebum;
- hairs;

- sebaceous glands;
- hair follicles;
- teeth;
- cartilage;
- gastrointestinal epithelium;
- nervous tissue;
- thyroid tissue.

Malignant change sometimes occurs in the form of squamous epithelioma or embryonal carcinoma in one of the elements of the tumour.

Hyperthyroidism may follow in a benign teratoma consisting mainly of thyroid tissue.

SOLID TERATOMA

This is a very rare tumour. It has a variety of primitive tissues with ectoderm, mesoderm and endoderm all represented so that the tumour consists of masses of embryonic cells of all varieties in a bizarre histological pattern. It is highly malignant.

CARCINOID TUMOUR

This is very rare in the ovary where it presents the same features as it does elsewhere in the body. These tumours are sometimes malignant.

GONADOBLASTOMA

This tumour occurs in abnormal gonads and in individuals who are sex chromatin negative. It consists of large germ cells like those of a dysgerminoma and small cells like granulosa cells. It may show hormonal activity and may become malignant.

GRANULOSA CELL TUMOUR

The cells resemble granulosa cells, being polygonal with deeply staining nuclei. They tend to be arranged in rosettes; clear space, Call-Exner bodies may be seen between them and strands of connective tissue run between the granulosa cells. Malignant change may occur.

Granulosa cell tumours may occur at any age. In infants and young children they are a rare cause of precocious puberty with uterine bleeding. In adult women, granulosa cell tumours cause profuse and irregular uterine bleeding from a hyperoestrogenized endometrium, often of metropathic type. An ovarian tumour must not be overlooked when considering these symptoms. In postmenopausal women irregular uterine bleeding is caused, with rejuvenation of the uterus, vulva and vagina. A hyperoestrogenized endometrium is found and there may be malignancy with associated carcinoma of the uterus.

THECOMA

This is a solid tumour which is usually 5 cm in diameter but may grow to 15 cm although this is rare. It resembles a fibroma and Meigs' syndrome can occur. Yellowish fatty areas which show up in sections stained for fat are scattered among the fibrous tissue cells. These are theca lutein cells. A mixed granulosa cell tumour and thecoma also occurs.

Thecoma occurs mainly in women over 30. It may present with a pelvic mass or with uterine haemorrhage or both; ascites and pleural effusions may be seen. There is a high incidence of carcinoma of the endometrium in association with thecoma.

ARRHENOBLASTOMA

Often called androblastoma, this tumour causes virilism from its testosterone metabolism but it is rare. The tumour may be cystic or solid and is potentially malignant. The cells consist of undifferentiated mesenchyme, and may be arranged in tubules as in the testicle.

CARCINOMA OF THE OVARY

Primary carcinoma of the ovary is the commonest malignant tumour found in gynaecology and an important cause of death in women, accounting for some 4500 deaths annually in England and Wales. It is a disease of middle and old age with 90% of cases in women above 45 years.

Risk factors relate to ovulatory history and the post activity of the germinal epithelium:
- increased risk—no pregnancy;
- decreased risk—many pregnancies—use of oral contraceptives.

Ovarian carcinoma may be cystic, arising usually from a benign cyst, or solid. Solid carcinoma may be papillary or an adenocarcinoma, undifferentiated carcinoma. It may arise in one of the special ovarian tumours such as granulosa cell tumour or dysgerminoma. Although accounting for only 1 to 2% of tumours, they are treatable using modern chemotherapy.

Spread of ovarian carcinoma

The main route of spread of carcinoma of the ovary is transcoelomically via the general peritoneal cavity, to the greater omentum and the peritoneum of the pouch of Douglas in particular. Ascites is frequent. Malignant tumours are often bilateral. Spread by lymphatics leads to involvement of the para-aortic glands; further spread may involve the supraclavicular glands. Blood-stream spread is unusual, death generally occurring from complications resulting from massive peritoneal secondaries.

METASTATIC OVARIAN TUMOURS

The ovary is a frequent site for secondary malignancy because of its rich blood supply. Adenocarcinoma is the commonest and the primary site may be the uterus, the other ovary, breast, stomach or large bowel. Secondary tumours in the ovary generally reproduce the cell structure of the primary growth.

STAGING CLASSIFICATION OF OVARIAN CARCINOMA

Stage I		**Tumour limited to the ovaries**
	IA	Tumour limited to one ovary
	IB	Tumour limited to both ovaries
	IC	IA or IB with capsule ruptured
		or
		surface involvement
		or
		malignant cells in ascites
		or
		peritoneal washings
Stage II		**Tumour involves one or both ovaries with pelvic spread**
	IIA	To tubes or uterus
	IIB	To other pelvic tissues
	IIC	IIA or IIB with malignant cells in ascites
		or
		peritoneal washings
Stage III		**Tumour involvement of abdominal cavity**
	IIIA	Microscopic peritoneal metastasis beyond pelvis
	IIIB	Macroscopic peritoneal metastasis $\leq 2\,cm$ diameter
		or
		involvement of retroperitoneal or inguinal nodes
	IIIC	Tumour in pelvis with involvement of small bowel
		or
		omentum
Stage IV		**Distant metastases**
		Liver
		Bowel
		Pleural fluid with malignant cells

Box 8.1 International Federation of Gynaecology and Obstetrics (FIGO) staging classification of ovarian carcinoma.

The *Krukenberg tumour* is an uncommon form of secondary carcinoma of the stomach or large bowel. The ovaries are enlarged by solid tumours, usually bilateral, which may reach 20 cm. Histologically they are characterized by the presence of signet ring cells which have undergone mucoid degeneration so that the nucleus is pushed to one side by a droplet of mucin.

Possibly a small number of Krukenberg tumours are primary in the ovary; patients have been known to survive for many years after removal of Krukenberg tumours with no primary tumour found at extensive investigation. This is not inconsistent with a microscopic slow-growing primary growth somewhere in the gastrointestinal tract which cures itself.

PAROVARIAN TUMOUR

This is not strictly a tumour of the ovary but is included for completeness since it presents clinically as an ovarian swelling. It is usually a unilocular cyst arising from a vestigial structure near the ovary or between the layers of the broad ligament. The cyst is lined with a single layer of cubical or columnar epithelium and contains clear serous fluid. Small polypoidal processes from the epithelium may project into the lumen of the tumour which is benign. It may reach a large size and be palpable up to or above the umbilicus. Because of its thin wall and its extraperitoneal situation in the broad ligament, surgical removal may present technical difficulties.

TREATMENT OF OVARIAN TUMOURS

The treatment of ovarian tumours is surgical removal as soon as the tumour is diagnosed with conservation of ovarian tissue in benign cases if possible. An exception may be made in the case of a cystic ovary which is less than 5 cm in diameter. Even if the tumour is apparently malignant and where ascites is present laparotomy should always be undertaken. Ascites may be associated with a benign tumour such as a fibroma, and even if there are metastases the prognosis is not hopeless. It may be possible to remove secondary masses in the omentum and if the primary tumour is removed, secondaries sometimes regress. An ovarian tumour, even if very large, is best removed intact. Tapping the fluid carries a risk of spilling the contents and contaminating the peritoneal cavity.

Small benign tumours can often be enucleated and the remaining normal ovary reconstructed at ovarian cystectomy; such conservative surgery is always advisable in women of childbearing age. This can be easily done laparoscopically with the right equipment and appropriate skill of the surgeon.

Carcinoma of the ovary should be treated initially by surgery which should involve total hysterectomy and bilateral salpingo-oophorectomy, though in young women a normal, uninvolved ovary might be left. In advanced cases, as much tissue as possible should be removed at a debulking operation and the greater omentum should be excised. A search should be made for peritoneal metastases, including those on the under surface of the diaphragm. A further second look laparotomy to ensure that the peritoneal cavity is free from secondary deposits may be carried out three to six months after the original operation.

Even in apparently advanced disease the ultimate prognosis appears to be improved by operative removal of the main tumour masses. The first operation offers the best chance to cure. It should be done by an experienced gynaecologist, preferably working in a specialist centre of gynaecologic oncology, who will do the widest excision with the least damage to ureters, bladder or intestines.

Radiotherapy is not much used in the management of ovarian cancer for it would have a deleterious affect on the bone marrow in the lumbar vertebrae and the liver.

Chemotherapy with cytotoxic agents gives more hopeful results and a variety have been or are under trial. Cisplatin, one of the platinum compounds gives good results, given in intravenous infusion and repeated every four weeks. Carboplatin is equally useful and has fewer side effects. In combination with other agents such as Taxane, the platinum compounds give a significant improvement result (see Box 8.2).

CHEMOTHERAPY TREATMENTS FOR OVARIAN CANCER

The general prognosis for ovarian carcinoma is poor, less than 20% surviving for five years. Factors which worsen prognosis are:

CHEMOTHERAPY WITH CYTOTOXIC AGENTS

Single alkylating agents
- Chlorambucil
- Melphalan
- Cyclophosphamide

Single platinum agents
- Cisplatin
- Carboplatin

Combinations
- Platinum agents plus cyclophosphamide
- Platinum agents plus cyclophosphamide plus doxorubicin

Box 8.2 Chemotherapy with Cytotoxic agents.

- advanced stage of disease;
- poorly differentiated tumour;
- how much tumour tissue remains after debulking surgery.

OVARIAN TUMOURS IN PREGNANCY

When a benign ovarian tumour is discovered in early pregnancy it is reasonable to defer operation until the 14th week, provided no urgent symptoms appear. The risk of abortion if operation is undertaken in the early weeks is greatly diminished after this stage of gestation.

A tumour discovered after the 28th week may also be left provided it is not thought to be malignant and is not likely to obstruct labour. It is best to await delivery and remove the tumour early in the puerperium. Caesarean section may have to be done if the tumour is obstructing descent of the fetus but should not be done mainly for the purpose of removing the ovarian mass.

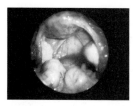

Disorders of menstruation

Amenorrhoea, 116
  Primary amenorrhoea, 116
  Genital agenesis, 116
Secondary amenorrhoea, 118
  Causes, 118
  Management, 120

Abnormal uterine bleeding, 122
  Menstrual variations, 122
  Intermittent bleeding, 122
Menorrhagia, 123
  Clinical course, 124
  Treatment of dysfunctional uterine bleeding, 125

Dysmenorrhoea, 130
  Spasmodic dysmenorrhoea, 130
  Secondary, congestive or acquired dysmenorrhoea, 132
Premenstrual tension, 132
Postmenopausal bleeding, 133

Menstruation is the discharge of blood from the uterus at approximately four-weekly intervals in women during the reproductive period; it is generally preceded by ovulation.

Menarche, the first menstruation, occurs at about 13 years of age, however, it may occur two to three years earlier or later; menstruation should be established by 17. At the onset, the cycle is often irregular and anovular cycles are common. At first bleeding is usually painless but may sometimes be prolonged.

Menstruation then continues until the menopause which usually occurs at about 50 but can occur between 35 to 55 years. Commonly the periods become more scanty, often with dark brown flow, and less frequent until they cease altogether. Profuse, prolonged or irregular bleeding are abnormal symptoms and demand full investigation.

About 60% of menopausal women experience hot flushes; vasomotor disturbances accompanied by a feeling of heat in the face and neck and sometimes sweating. They may occur as frequently as four times a day. Some women are very distressed by them while others hardly notice. Nervous tension and irritability tend to occur at this time and many women gain weight. For some, however, the menopause is a blessing as it marks the end of childbearing.

Many women experience symptoms of abdominal or pelvic pain during the menstrual cycle at the time of ovulation due to peritoneal irritation from the release of follicular fluid; this is known as *mittelschmerz*. In the luteal phase of menstruation there may be retention of fluid with corresponding weight gain and sometimes detectable oedema. The breasts may become tense and tender and the waist measurement may increase. Psychological irritability with depression and emotional instability can occur, the premenstrual tension syndrome. These symptoms may be relieved after a day or two of menstruation but during the menses many women feel off colour.

Anovular menstruation occurs especially in the first year of menses in young girls, for a few years before menopause and also after childbirth. Follicles develop but there is no ovulation and so no corpus luteum; bleeding then takes place from a proliferative endometrium following oestrogen stimulation unregulated by progesterone. Anovular bleeding is generally painless.

AMENORRHOEA

Primary amenorrhoea

Menstruation not begun by the age of 17 must be distinguished from cryptomenorrhoea—hidden loss caused by obstruction to menstrual flow. This is most often caused by a septum across the vagina just above the hymen. On inspection of the vulva a bluish bulge is seen just inside the hymen. There may be cyclical attacks of abdominal pain and a mass may be palpable *per abdomen*, representing a large haematocolpos and a haematoma as well.

TREATMENT

Incise the septum and express the haematocolpos by suprapubic pressure. Take care to avoid infection. If none occurs, subsequent menstruation and childbearing are normal.

CAUSES OF PRIMARY AMENORRHOEA

- Physiological amenorrhoea occurs before puberty.
- Psychogenic, hypothalamic or environmental amenorrhoea may follow a severe emotional shock or a change in climate.
- Common in girls who leave home for the first time; it is often seen in students. Spontaneous recovery is the rule.

Genital agenesis

There may be primary agenesis of the ovaries, e.g., Turner's syndrome, or agenesis or hypoplasia of the uterus.

INVESTIGATION OF PRIMARY AMENORRHOEA

A *history* is taken including a family history as testicular feminization may affect other females in the family.

Physical examination. The general examination should begin by recording the girl's height—if by 16 she is less than 147 cm there is a possibility of ovarian agenesis (Turner's syndrome) or panhypopituitarism. If there is an increase in body weight, calculate Ponderal Index. A general examination checks the development of secondary sexual characteristics, hair patterns and density.

A *Pelvic examination* should be performed if the examiner really thinks a positive finding will be there. For most young women with primary amenorrhoea it will be not useful particularly at first consultation. The vulva is inspected to see that the introitus is patent; there may be cryptomenorrhoea, congenital absence of the vagina or a blind vagina as in testicular feminization.

Investigations. A buccal smear and an examination of the polymorphonuclear leucocytes to determine if chromatin positive (probably XX) or chromatin negative (probably XO or XY); in doubtful cases a full chromosome analysis may be needed to exclude mosaicism.

If there are virilizing changes, excretion of 17-oxosteroids will be raised in cases of congenital or acquired adrenogenital syndrome; the dexamethasone suppression test will exclude an adrenal tumour. Further investigations of hormone levels may be required on obscure cases.

Ultrasound will help determine the presence, state and size of the ovaries and any follicular activity. Uterine size can also be seen. It is rarely necessary to perform a laparoscopy to assess the pelvic organs and take an ovarian biopsy.

MANAGEMENT

If the girl is normally developed, with normal breast development, the uterus and vagina are normal and she is chromatin positive, the most likely diagnosis is delayed menarche. It is reasonable to await events; menstruation is not established in some individuals before 20 years. There is little point in giving hormones to induce uterine cyclical bleeding as they may inhibit ovulation.

If the girl is anxious, a trial of three month's stimulation of ovulation with clomiphene will reassure her but do not go on stimulating; keep the therapy in reserve until she needs the oocytes for ovulation and pregnancy.

For those with a diagnosable pathological cause, the aim must be to restore normal function as far as possible and although fertility may not be possible, enable the individual to lead as normal a sexual life as possible.

Cases of Turner's syndrome often have no breast development, a webbed neck, a wide carrying angle at the elbows and they may have coarctation of the aorta; they are XO, chromatin negative. They should receive long-term treatment with cyclical hormones, oestrogen and progestogen. There is a small risk of uterine carcinoma.

In testicular feminization, the gonad is a testis which secretes an oestrogen due to a fault in testosterone receptors. The abnormal gonad, which may be in an inguinal hernia, should be removed and after puberty an artificial vagina may be constructed to permit sexual intercourse. Treatment with oestrogen and progesterone may also be given though there will be no menstruation.

In cases of congenital absence of the vagina and uterus the ovaries are usually normal. An artificial vagina may be constructed to permit sexual intercourse.

The androgenital syndrome is treated with cortisone and normal function and fertility may ensue; adrenal tumours are potentially malignant and should be removed.

Abnormalities of pituitary secretion should be treated.

SECONDARY AMENORRHOEA

Causes

PHYSIOLOGY

Amenorrhoea occurs in:
- pregnancy;
- lactation;
- after menopause.

PSYCHOLOGY

- A great desire for pregnancy.
- A great fear and dread of pregnancy.

PITUITARY

Simmond's disease follows total pituitary ablation or destruction by radiotherapy. Tumours may also destroy it. In Sheehan's syndrome, severe postpartum haemorrhage causes pituitary anoxia with failure of lactation, amenorrhoea and other manifestations of pituitary failure. In the Chiari-Frommel syndrome, again after postpartum haemorrhage, there is amenorrhoea galactorrhoea and an excess prolactin secretion. Hyperprolactinaemia may also follow a definitive pituitary adenoma or scattered microadenoma.

Anorexia nervosa may lead to pituitary damage and thus to permanent amenorrhoea and sterility. Periods cease before weight loss becomes apparent.

The adrenogenital syndrome may be congenital or acquired after adrenal hyperplasia or tumour. There is virilism with amenorrhoea. The excretion of 17-oxosteroids is increased with a low cortisol output.

THYROID DISEASE

Hyperthyroidism tends to cause amenorrhoea, but all thyroid disorders may case amenorrhoea or excessive bleeding. Correction of the thyroid function may restore normal menstruation.

OTHER CAUSES

Spontaneous premature ovarian failure in the absence of disease causes premature menopause. The ovary ceases to respond to pituitary gonadotrophin which may be excreted in excessive amounts or may be normal. This follows a lack of oocytes.

Castration by surgical removal of the ovaries or by exposure to irradiation leads to amenorrhoea.

Extensive destruction of the ovaries by infection or tumours is a rare cause.

Arrhenoblastoma leads to virilism with amenorrhoea.

Polycystic ovary syndrome consists of stromal hyperplasia of the ovaries, leading to thickening of the tunica albuginea and the formation of multiple follicular cysts; it is associated with obesity, amenorrhoea, hirsutism and infertility.

UTERINE

The endometrium is destroyed by several means:
- By disease:
    (a) tuberculosis;
    (b) severe postpartum infection.
- By formal endometrial ablation.
- By severe curettage.

GENERAL DISEASE

Amenorrhoea may occur in any debilitating disease, e.g., pulmonary tuberculosis; not necessarily with involvement of the pelvic organs.

Terminal stages of diseases such as Addison's disease and uraemia due to renal disease.

Starvation may lead to amenorrhoea, similar to that seen in anorexia nervosa.

Obesity can also cause amenorrhoea, and in grossly obese young women weight reduction may restore normal menstrual function.

Management

Secondary amenorrhoea is physiological during pregnancy, lactation and at the menopause. A premature menopause may occur as early as 35 years of age. Significant amenorrhoea in the absence of physiological causes is the absence of menstruation for 12 months. However, women get very concerned about this symptom and will often request investigation and treatment before this.

HISTORY

- Family history.
- Hot flushes.
- Drugs such as resperine, digoxin, phenothiazines and hormones, including oral contraceptives.
- Change in body weight i.e., obesity or sudden loss of weight.
- A few women with secondary amenorrhoea are cases of primary amenorrhoea who have had withdrawal bleeding following ill-advised attempts to induce menstruation with hormones.

PHYSICAL EXAMINATION

- Height measurement.
- Weight.
- Blood pressure.
- Secondary sexual characteristics.
- Breasts for evidence of pregnancy or milk secretion.
- Pelvic examination to:
   (a) exclude pregnancy (a woman may conceive in the course of a period of amenorrhoea);
   (b) assess the size and position of the uterus to exclude a pelvic tumour.

INVESTIGATIONS

- X-ray of the chest and the pituitary fossa; if relevant, CT scan of pituitary area.
- Glucose tolerance test.
- Thyroid function tests.
- Thyroxine, T3 binding index.
- Free-thyroxine index. Thyroid stimulating hormone (TSH).

- 24-hour urine for 17-oxosteroids.
- Dexamethasone suppression test.
- Plasma hormone levels of follicle stimulating hormone (FSH).
- Luteinizing hormone.
- Oestradiol.
- Prolactin.

These should be repeated at weekly intervals for four weeks to assess ovarian and pituitary function.

Ultrasound assessment of:

- uterine size;
- pregnancy in uterus;
- ovarian size;
- follicular function.

Rarely examination under anaesthesia to:

- assess the pelvic organs;
- assess the ovaries;
- measure the uterine cavity;
- perform a laparoscopy to inspect the pelvic organs and to take a biopsy of the ovaries.

TREATMENT

Treat the cause if one is discovered. Treatment will depend on whether fertility is desired or not.

In *hypothalamic* amenorrhoea, spontaneous return of normal menstruation occurs in the majority in 6 to 18 months.

In *anorexia nervosa* the periods may cease before weight loss is evident; treatment should include efforts to restore weight to normal. In *gross obesity*, weight loss may result in normal menstruation.

In cases where there is anxiety and where amenorrhoea has persisted for many months, especially after stopping the contraceptive pill, treatment may be justified to stimulate the restart of ovulation. Give clomiphene citrate in a dose of 50 mg daily for five days for three cycles. Often there is a response and normal menstruation continues.

A *premature menopause* is characterized by low oestrogen levels and high FSH. They may improve by artificially induced menstruation with a preparation of cyclical oestrogen and progesterone such as Cyclo-Progynova.

Where excess of prolactin (about 1000 μu/l) is secreted, perform a CT scan of the pituitary fossa to exclude a tumour. In the absence of such a space occupying lesion, microadenoma of the pituitary body are postulated. Treatment of amenorrhoea with prolactin excess is with bromocriptine 2.5 mg daily for three days; then 2.5 mg twice a day for six months.

Cases of *sterility with amenorrhoea* require complex investigation and treatment; those who do not respond to clomiphene require treatment under careful hormone control with gonadotrophins.

In the *polycystic ovary syndrome* partial resection of the ovaries has proved disappointing, but laparoscopically directed needle diathermy may be helpful. Cortisone (prednisone) is preferred in this condition. Clomiphene is also useful to stimulate follicular maturation.

Hypomenorrhoea (scanty loss at the periods) and *oligomenorrhoea* (infrequent periods) are caused by many of the conditions which cause secondary amenorrhoea; the investigation and treatment are the same.

ABNORMAL UTERINE BLEEDING

Menstrual variations

There are many Latin words to describe abnormal bleeding. It is probably better to use Anglo-Saxon and describe the symptoms as *heavy periods* or *prolonged periods* but the classic terms are still in use and need definition.

- *Menorrhagia* is an excessive loss of blood with regular menstruation.
- *Metrorrhagia* is prolonged bleeding from the uterus.
- *Metro-menorrhagia* is heavy and prolonged periods.
- *Polymenorrhoea* is frequent menstruation.

These may be associated with *complications of early and undiagnosed pregnancy.*

- Abortion.
- Ectopic pregnancy.
- Hydatidiform mole.

Foreign bodies in the uterus — intrauterine contraceptives.

Treatment with hormones especially in menopausal and post-menopausal women. Breakthrough bleeding may occur with synthetic progestogens given for oral contraception or for treatment of pelvic disorders.

Psychosomatic causes, for example a severe emotional shock, may induce irregular bleeding.

An abnormal bleeding tendency may be present such as leukaemia or Hodgkin's disease.

Hyper- or hypothyroidism may be associated with menorrhagia or irregular bleeding.

Intermittent bleeding

The causes of non-cyclical abnormal vaginal bleeding not associated with menstruation include:

- *lesions of the cervix*—polypi; carcinoma; vascular erosion;
- *lesions of the body of the uterus*—endometritis; fibroids; polypi; adenomyosis; carcinoma; sarcoma.

The level of haemoglobin is generally lower in women than in men between the ages of 15 and 50; this difference is accounted for by blood loss and the consequent iron deficiency associated with menstruation and childbearing. Menorrhagia or metrorrhagia can lead to anaemia but many women with true heavy loss are able to respond to the chronic repeated demand on their bone marrow. Older women are less able to do this.

MENORRHAGIA

The range of normal menstrual loss is 10 to 60 ml per cycle. If above 80 ml, this is considered excessive. More commonly, diagnosis is made on the woman's history:

- increase in the number of pads or tampons used to more than 10 per day;
- starting to pass clots in the menstrual flow;
- use of a pictorial blood loss assessment chart which gives a semi-quantitative measure of loss (Fig. 3.5).

Up to 30% of women in the later part of menstrual life complain of heavy periods. Only a half of these actually lose more than 80 ml of blood per period. The diagnosis, however, rests on the woman's history rather than scientific measurement.

AETIOLOGY

Menorrhagia commonly is a presenting symptom in:
- fibroids;
- endometriosis;
- pelvic inflammatory disease;
- incorrectly controlled hormone therapy (including oral contraception).

Less commonly, it is associated with:
- endometrial polypi;
- an intrauterine device (IUD);
- recent tubal ligation;
- functional ovarian tumours;
- disorders of clotting (e.g., von Willebrand's disease).

Menorrhagia is not caused by:
- anticoagulation of the woman for antithrombotic reasons;
- idiopathic thrombocytopenic purpura.

After full examination and investigation (including a D&C) in about 50% of women with true menorrhagia, no obvious pathology is found.

This is *dysfunctional uterine haemorrhage* implicating a malfunction of the endocrine controlling systems. A better name would be *menorrhagia of unknown origin*.

Clinical course

While menorrhagia is most commonly found in the over 35-year-old, it can occur at any stage in female life up to the menopause. The causes and management may be classified according to age group.

BIRTH TO 18 YEARS OF AGE

Female infants may have vaginal bleeding during the first week of life. This is rarely significant and probably due to withdrawal of maternally derived oestrogens which had crossed the placenta in pregnancy.

Precocious puberty is caused by premature maturation of the ovaries in most cases; very rarely there may be a granulosa cell tumour of the ovary (Chapter 8). The breasts swell while pubic and axillary hair develop and endometrial bleeding occurs; sometimes with ovulation. Provided a tumour of the ovary can be excluded, the child may be allowed to develop normally but the parents must be warned of the danger of pregnancy.

The differential diagnosis includes:
• a mixed mesodermal tumour;
• adenocarcinoma of the vagina; particularly at risk were adolescent girls whose mothers received stilboestrol during pregnancy but this is now history.

Adolescent bleeding of a sufficient amount to be considered as menorrhagia is usually dysfunctional. There may be prolonged episodes of painless bleeding and the girl may become anaemic. Examination of the endometrium may show an anovulatory pattern or hyperplasia.

Treatment consists of eliminating any organic cause and correcting anaemia if present. Hormone treatment is usually successful using an oestrogen, such as ethinyloestradiol 0.05 mg daily begun on the fifth day of an episode of bleeding; the dose may be increased to stop bleeding. After 10 days a progesterone such as norethisterone is added in a dose of 15 mg daily for 10 days, the oestrogen being continued during this time. When the treatment is stopped, withdrawal bleeding with shedding of the endometrium (a medical curettage) analogous with normal menstruation occurs. Treatment should be given for a further three to six months. After treatment is stopped, menstruation is often normal. In cases where this fails, curettage should be performed.

WOMEN AGED 18 TO 40 YEARS

In this group true dysfunctional bleeding is uncommon and the most likely cause of abnormal bleeding is some complication of pregnancy. Occasionally heavier periods follow tubal ligation for sterilization. Diagnostic curettage is rarely needed in this group for the possibility of malignant disease is unusual.

WOMEN AGED OVER 35

All the organic causes of bleeding, including malignant disease, may occur and it is essential to exclude them.

Among women without organic disease, three main patterns of the endometrium are seen on histological examination.

• *Atrophic*, with bleeding occurring by a seepage through the thin lining of the uterus.

• A *mixed pattern* with proliferative and secretory endometrium with possibly endometrial polypi. This is associated with irregular shedding of the endometrium for the normal mechanism of ovulation and so menstruation is disordered so the endometrium is not completely shed.

• *Hyperplasia* of the endometrium may involve the glands or the stroma or both. *Cystic hyperplasia* (metropathia haemorrhagica) is common in menopausal women. There is usually amenorrhoea followed by prolonged bleeding from the hyper-oestrogenized endometrium. The ovaries contain many follicular cysts. A similar pattern is seen with an oestrogen secreting tumour or feminizing mesenchymoma of the ovary (Chapter 8). There is no great risk of cystic hyperplasia going on to carcinoma of the endometrium. Atypical hyperplasia is more likely to be associated with endometrial carcinoma, the risk depending on the degree of the atypia.

Treatment of dysfunctional uterine bleeding

Treatment should never be given without accurate diagnosis except perhaps in girls under 18 with puberty bleeding. Blind hormone treatment is particularly dangerous as malignant disease may be masked.

DIAGNOSIS

Investigation should include an endometrial biopsy. This may be done in the out-patients department using:

• a suction curette (Fig. 9.1);
• a small biopsy loop (Fig. 9.2).

With appropriate skills, passing these causes little discomfort, about the same as fitting an IUD. This avoids admission and the general anaesthetic for a D&C. However, a fuller curettage is indicated if:

• it is impossible to pass the curette because of a tight cervix;
• the woman is anxious and cannot relax;

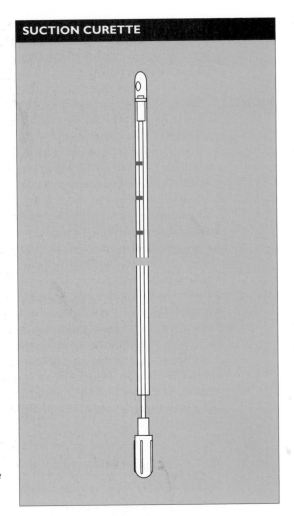

SUCTION CURETTE

Fig. 9.1 A suction curette for out-patient biopsy of the endometrium.

• there is a high risk of malignancy of the endometrium.

Hysteroscopy may accompany the curettage in the out-patients department if the gynaecologist is skilled and properly equipped. It is excellent at showing endometrial polyps and submucous fibroids which could be missed by blind curettage. In many cases an organic diagnosis will be made and appropriate treatment be given.

DRUG THERAPY

This is the first line of treatment because it:

• is more convenient, being administered in the out-patients department or GP surgery;

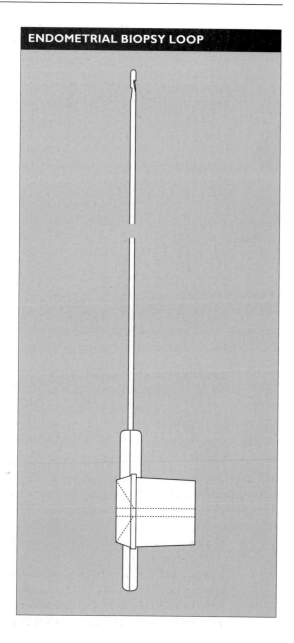

ENDOMETRIAL BIOPSY LOOP

Fig. 9.2 An endometrial biopsy loop for outpatient use.

- avoids surgery with general anaesthesia;
- retains the uterus, a major factor for some women;
- is much cheaper:
    - (a) in finance to the Health Authority or Trust;

(b) in time (and therefore maybe finance) to the woman.

Treatment may be non-hormonal or hormonal (see Boxes 9.1 and 9.2).

NON-HORMONAL TREATMENT

Taken during menses, hence no problem if accidental pregnancy is present

Prostaglandin synthetase inhibitors
Reduce uterine prostaglandins
Mefenamic acid   500 mg six hourly during menstruation of 12 to
                  18 months
                  Avoid if peptic ulceration
Fenamates

Antifibrinolytic Agents
Reduce abnormal fibrinolysis
Avoid if history of thrombosis
Tranexamic acid   1 g six hourly during menstruation
Ethamsylate   500 mg four hourly during menstruation

Box 9.1 Non-hormonal treatment.

HORMONAL TREATMENT

This aims at imitating or restoring the normal endocrine cycle

Norethisterone   5 mg three times a day from Day 15 to
                  Day 26 of cycle for six to nine months.
                  If no cycle, plan one with the calendar.
                  Progestogen; best for those with anovular cycles
                  Cheap and good for emergency treatment:
                  10 mg three times a day for very heavy
                  bleeding

Danazol   200 mg daily continuously for three to six months
                  Derivative of testosterone so
                  antioestrogenic – at hypothalamus
                                  – at endometrium
                  Expensive. May be weight gain and androgenization

Oral contraceptive – Dose according to brand but probably best to use
                    cyclical combined oestrogen (30 μg) and
                    progestogen (0.25 mg)
                    Practical, cheap & easily available

Box 9.2 Hormonal treatment.

SURGICAL THERAPY

Based on removal of the endometrium or the uterus with its endometrium.

Curettage

- Removes outer layers of endometrium but leaves the basal layers from which new tissue arises in a month or so.
- Ineffective treatment—one or two menses may be less heavy but are soon back to previous level or heavier.

Cryotherapy

- Liquid nitrogen probes ($-180°C$) applied through the cervix under anaesthetic destroy endometrium down to myometrium.
- Not very effective in the long term because blind application allows a lot of endometrium to remain. This spreads laterally and within months menstruation is as heavy as before.

Transcervical ablation

- Under vision through a hysteroscope, endometrium is destroyed:
    - (a) with electrocoagulating loops;
    - (b) with a laser.
- At present, needs general anaesthesia but this is a much smaller procedure, upsetting patient less and requiring only one day in hospital:
    - (a) uterus retained although lining (mostly) gone;
    - (b) after a year, 30% have amenorrhoea and another 60% report lighter blood loss;
    - (c) if it fails (10 to 20%), can proceed to either repeat ablation or to hysterectomy.
- It is not a little operation:
    - (a) requires manipulative skills;
    - (b) requires expensive equipment;
    - (c) risks of perforating uterus (1%);
    - (d) risks of artery damage and bleeding (less than 1%);
    - (e) risks of damaging bowel (less than 1%).
- However, save of time and hospital stay:
    - (a) early return to normal activity;
    - (b) keeping uterus makes it popular;
    - (c) contraception is still required unless there is complete amenorrhoea.

Hysterectomy

- Removal of the uterus stops periods.

Abdominal hysterectomy
- Major procedure with general anaesthesia.
- Abdominal scar to heal.
- Hospital stay 4 to 6 days.
- Risks of damage to ureters.
- Risks of damage to the bladder.
- Risks of damage to the bowel.

Vaginal hysterectomy
- Needs to be a mobile, adhesion free uterus.
- Need small uterus.
- Helps if there is some prolapse.

Laparoscopy assisted hysterectomy
- Smaller abdominal incision.
- Needs skilled laparoscopic surgeon.
- Does the difficult part of a vaginal hysterectomy from above ligating tubes, ovarian suspensory ligament and round ligament via laparoscopy. Then an easy vaginal removal.
- Has all the complications of laparoscopy surgery.

    Hysterectomy does not have to be accompanied by removal of ovaries.

Indications for oophorectomy
- If ovaries abnormal.
- If family history of ovarian cancer.
- If over 50 years old.
    Retain:
- if menses cycling regularly;
- if ovaries healthy at surgery.

DYSMENORRHOEA

Dysmenorrhoea or pain associated with menstruation occurs in two main forms:
- primary spasmodic;
- secondary, congestive or acquired.

Spasmodic dysmenorrhoea

This is very common; most normal women have some discomfort at the onset of menstruation. In dysmenorrhoea, pain is severe during the first hours or days of the period. It may be:

- continuous or spasmodic like colic;
- accompanied by vomiting and fainting;
- felt in the pelvis and lower back;
- radiating into the legs.

It does not begin at the onset of menstruation when the cycles are often anovular, and it is commonest in single women or infertile married women. It tends to lessen after the age of 25 and to disappear after 30.

CAUSE

The pain is probably caused by ischaemia after the powerful contractions of the uterine muscle in the first days of menstruation. There is rarely any pathological cause found.

Some women with primary dysmenorrhoea have a lowered threshold for pain, possibly caused by emotional disturbance or boredom with monotonous work. Childbirth often cures the condition, possibly because the parous uterus is more vascular and does not become so ischaemic.

MANAGEMENT

May be summed up as follows:

- Attention to general health. Menstrual hygiene is important and a hot bath or shower should be taken daily during menstruation.
- Simple analgesics. Aspirin, paracetamol and codeine or combination of these may be used. Mefenamic acid (500 mg three times a day) gives good relief of pain in many cases. Phenacetin should be avoided because of the risk of kidney damage; amphetamines may lead to addiction and should be avoided. For this reason morphine and pethidine should also be avoided however severe the pain may seem to be.
- Hormone treatment includes oral contraception to inhibit ovulation and thus cause painless bleeding. One of the low-dose oral contraceptives may be preferred though women sometimes object to contraceptives being given so they are called menstrual regulants. The best effect follows hormones that inhibit ovulation. Given for a few months at a time they cause no ill effects and improvement may continue when treatment is stopped perhaps because of increased vascularity in the uterus.
- Dilatation of the cervix is a traditional treatment which gives relief in some cases, though often only temporarily. Do not over dilate the cervix for this may cause incompetence of the internal os and consequent recurrent abortions.
- Presacral resection may be performed in intractable cases but is rarely required.

Secondary, congestive or acquired dysmenorrhoea

This is rare before 25 years and uncommon before 30.

SYMPTOMS

Pain begins before menstruation and may be relieved when bleeding starts. It is felt in the pelvis and back and made worse with exertion. Other symptoms such as menorrhagia and dyspareunia may be present.

This type of dysmenorrhoea usually occurs with a physical cause.

- Chronic pelvic sepsis (Chapter 11).
- Endometriosis (Chapter 12).
- Acquired fixed retroversion of the uterus.
- Fibroids.

PREMENSTRUAL TENSION

Premenstrual tension occurs most usually in the second half of menstrual life. It consists of a cluster of behavioural symptoms to physical signs which come in the second half of the cycle with abolition immediately after menstruation.

SYMPTOMS AND SIGNS

- Irritability.
- Depression.
- Lassitude.
- Insomnia.
- Lack of concentration.
- Oedema with fluid retention.
- Abdominal swelling.
- Swollen fingers and ankles.
- Weight gain.

Migraine can occur during this phase or at the onset of menstruation. The symptoms tend to come on 7 to 10 days premenstrually, after the luteal phase is established. Women may become more accident prone and there is an increased prevalence of suicide. Some women who suffer from premenstrual tension have endogenous depression exacerbated at this time.

AETIOLOGY

Genetic
- Commoner in monozygotic twins than dizygotic.

Psychological
- A possible association with neuroticism.

Hormonal
- Timing in cycle in luteal phase.
- Improved in absence of cyclical ovarian activity.
- Renin–angiotensin system.
- Reduction of endogenous opioids.
- Changes in mono-amine neurotransmitters.
  Probably a combination of the second and third factors.

TREATMENT

- Explanation and reassurance.
- Diuretics such as frusemide 20 to 40 mg daily for three days at a time may be given if oedema a problem.
- Progestogens—may be deficient in second half of cycle so replace them.
- Oestrogens—to suppress ovulation.
- Oral contraceptive—combined preparation of both of the above; works for a few.
- Prostaglandin synthetase inhibitors—mefenamic acid helps some.
- Danazol—stops ovulation; beware unwanted androgenic side effects.
- GnRH—reduces ovarian function; works for some.
- Evening primrose oil—may effect essential fatty acid metabolism.
- Pyridoxine (B$_6$)—may affect dopamine and serotonin metabolism. Benefit weak—beware over dosage and neuropathy with long-term treatment.
- Anti-depressants—during the premenstrual phase may help. More severe cases need psychiatric treatment.

  The variety of medication emphasizes how little the cause of this syndrome is understood. Treatments may be a matter of trial and error.

POSTMENOPAUSAL BLEEDING

Postmenopausal bleeding is bleeding from the genital tract occurring six months or more after the menopause. It is a serious symptom which may indicate the presence of malignant disease in the genital tract. Every woman with postmenopausal bleeding should be assumed to have a carcinoma until a full investigation has proved to the contrary.

The chief causes are:

The vulva
- Carcinoma.

- Urethral caruncle.
  Rectal bleeding and haematuria must be excluded.

The vagina
- Carcinoma.
- Vaginitis, especially atrophic vaginitis.
- Foreign bodies, especially pessaries.

The cervix
- Carcinoma of the ectocervix.
- Carcinoma of a cervical canal polyp.

The endometrium
- Carcinoma.
- Sarcoma.
- Mixed mesodermal tumours.
- Polyp.
- Atrophic endometritis.

The fallopian tube
- Carcinoma.

The ovary
- Feminizing tumours.
- Granulosa cell tumour.
- Theca cell tumour.

HORMONE TREATMENT

Withdrawal bleeding may follow administration of oestrogens for menopausal symptoms. This should not be assumed to be the cause of any postmenopausal bleeding until a full investigation including cytology and curettage has excluded more sinister causes.

CHAPTER 10

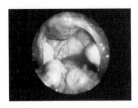

The menopause

Physiology, 135
   Symptoms, 136
   Other symptoms, 137
   Long-term symptoms,
      137

Postmenopausal therapy,
   137
Long-term therapy,
   139

Complications of
   hormone replacement
   therapy, 140
Premature menopause, 141

The menopause is the cessation of normal menstruation. The climacteric is a longer period during which time the reproductive organs involute. These time zones overlap each other in time just as they do in youth with the two processes of menarche and puberty.

The mean age of menopause is 51 with a normal range from 45 to 56. Conventionally a woman has to stop menstruating for six months before she is considered to be postmenopausal.

PHYSIOLOGY

At the end of reproductive life, the ovaries become less able to produce oocytes due to:
- a lack of primordial follicles, because all have been used;
- more refractory receptor function in the granulosa and thecal cells.

Hence, the production of FSH is greatly increased from the pituitary in order to stimulate the failing ovaries still more. The failing oestrogen levels do not stimulate the endometrium to produce the follicular phase which starts the cycle. The lack of progesterone does not allow organization of the endometrium to form a luteal phase of the cycle.

The ovarian stroma produces androstenedione which converts in peripheral fat to oestrone, a weaker oestrogen than oestradiol, the steroid on which the woman has depended on for much of her reproductive life. Menstruation stops due to a lack of cyclical oestrogen and progesterone stimulation. The low sensitivity of the bones of the body to the reabsorbing effects of the parathyroid hormones is increased in the presence of low oestrogen levels. Hence, the bones of some women become osteoporotic.

Symptoms

At the menopause 60% of women are relatively asymptomatic, 25% of women have mild symptoms and 15% have moderate to severe symptoms. The two commonest symptoms are:

- hot flushes;
- dryness of the vagina.

There is often a loss of libido; part is hormonal but much is psychogenic.

Mood swings, nervousness, anxiety, irritability and depression are all measured in this group of women. The decrease of oestrogens may reduce their modulatory role on brain mono-amine synthesis, but many social changes occur in a family at this time such as the departure of children.

Symptoms are found more commonly in those who had premenstrual tension or dysmenorrhoea. The symptoms are less frequent in Asian and Negro women, possibly associated with the removal of menstrual taboos in their societies or the loss of fertility among a group who use contraception less frequently.

HOT FLUSHES

These are the feeling of heat over the face and upper part of the body usually lasting for half to one minute. They are followed by perspiration of this area, which may render the woman wringing wet. These flushes usually last for a year or so and in up to a quarter of women at least four years. This is probably due to an increase in the sympathetic nervous system drive mediated through the central neurotransmitters. They come on more at night when in bed and can wake a woman up.

DRY VAGINA

Secretions from the cervix and the surface glands are diminished and the vaginal epithelium becomes thinner, less elastic with a reduced blood supply; atrophic vaginitis follows. Lower oestrogen levels alter these oestrogen dependent tissues. Dryness and, therefore, dyspareunia is common. Intercourse should not be attempted unless there is adequate extra lubrication available.

The labia tend to lose their fat and so the vagina becomes more exposed to the outside world, particularly when sitting down on a hard surface.

OTHER GENITAL CHANGES

The breasts become atrophic and the nipples flatten. The uterus becomes smaller. There is less support from the cardinal ligament, utero-sacral and the utero pubic ligaments so support in the pelvis is more precarious.

Other symptoms

The lower oestrogen levels lead to atrophy of the urethra causing frequency of micturition, dysuria and urgency (urethral syndrome). The weakness of the supporting muscles and the cardinal ligaments allow stress incontinence to start at this age.

The pulling back of the posterior wall of the urethra often exposes the sensitive anterior wall which becomes inflamed. A small polyp may occur on the posterior wall or a urethral caruncle.

The reduction of oestrogens allows a release in the levels of high density lipoproteins, cholesterol and triglycerides. This is accompanied by a catch-up rate for women of coronary heart disease.

Long-term symptoms

Most of the above symptoms disappear within a year or two but those on the skeleton stay for ever.

The calcium part of the skeleton is reabsorbed, whilst the collagen framework stays the same. This leads to osteoporosis. Bone reabsorption is worse when calcium intake is low, though it is not greatly diminished when calcium intake is high. Continued osteoporosis leads to fractures of the neck of the femur and the wrist. Compression fractures at the front of the vertebrae occur in about a quarter of women a decade after the menopause.

Women lose calcium at different rates and so the need for replacement oestrogens differs from one woman to another. If they are given at the same time as a poor calcium diet they are less effective. In reproductive life, while oestrogen synthesis is high, women are greatly protected from heart disease and coronary occlusion. After the menopause, this does not occur and ten years later, the rate of coronary thrombosis is as high in women as men. Although at present not well understood, this coronary artery protection effect may be an important reason for hormone replacement treatment (HRT) (Fig. 10.1).

POSTMENOPAUSAL THERAPY

The treatment for postmenopausal symptoms is:

1 the acute oestrogen replacement for women who have symptoms, principally hot flushes and dry vagina;

2 the more chronic replacement therapy for women who are losing

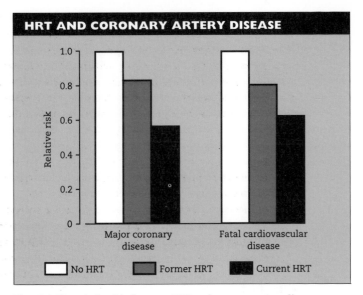

Fig. 10.1 The relationship between HRT and coronary artery disease.

oestrogen in order to prevent osteoporosis and reduce the incidence of coronary heart disease.

The giving of symptomatic oestrogen replacement is the more straightforward therapy. The only contra-indication, if a woman has symptoms, is a history of breast cancer or endometrial cancer.

The aim should be to use the lowest effective dose of oestrogen for the shortest period of time. It is usual to give it in a cyclical fashion of 21 or 28 days. This causes remission of symptoms in most women, once the correct dose is achieved.

Progestogens are added in the second half of the cycle to enhance the shedding of the endometrium and so prevent a build up of endometrium with possible hyperplasia, or atypical hyperplasia and then malignancy.

Owing to the cyclical nature of the treatment, the endometrium which develops during the oestrogen phase is shed after withdrawal and so there appears to be a continuation of menstrual periods.

The hormone may be given in a number of ways, as described below.

Orally

This is the commonest and the most convenient. Compliance may be patchy and patients may forget, rendering the therapy ineffective.

Transdermal patches
Oestrogen and progestogens are readily absorbed through the skin. There is the advantage of the oestrogen not having to pass through the portal system after absorption, where much would be destroyed. Hence, higher tissue levels of the oestrogens are achieved. Skin reactions may occur in up to 20% of patients (blistering and hyperaemia). The patches only need to be changed every third day and so compliance is higher.

Implants
Oestrogens can be given in a retard preparation by implantation under local anaesthesia. The pellets can be inserted into the abdominal wall or the thigh under the fascia lata. They last four to eight months and are easily replaced so compliance is not relevant. Usually the oestrogens are given with testosterone to provide some stimulus to the libido.

Progesterones should be taken by mouth during the second half of each cycle in order to get a withdrawal bleed and prevent build-up of the endometrium.

Vaginally
Steroids are absorbed through the vaginal epithelium but a large dose is needed in the vagina to get a reasonable dose inside the body. However, if vaginal dryness is the main symptom, this is a good route.

PREPARATIONS

1 Orally – Progynova, oestradiol or Premarin (oestrone). Progestogen – norethisterone 1 mg a day for last 10 days.
2 Sub-cutaneous implant – 100 mg oestradiol with 100 mg testosterone.
3 Patches of oestradiol 25 or 50 μg with norethisterone acetate 1 mg.
4 Vaginal application – oestriol or oestradiol as a cream or pessary high in the vagina once a day.

All treatments should be given for between six and eighteen months. If the uterus has been removed previously, the supplementary progesterone is not required. Unless treatment is stopped for an interval, the doctor and the patient will never know if the treatment is still required.

Long-term therapy

This is replacement therapy for the absence of oestrogen. It should be looked upon the same way as insulin is given to diabetics.

Whilst this was originally given to prevent osteoporosis, there is much evidence now that it could reduce the incidence of coronary heart disease by as much as 40% in women in the postmenopausal era; this is probably due to the effect of oestrogens on blood lipids combined with a depressant effect on blood platelets and on increased blood flow.

Bone densimetry, where the amount of calcium in bone is checked physically, is not precise enough to provide an effective screening test for the risk of fractures. Hence, it is not good enough to check which women might need hormone replacement therapy for the prevention of osteoporosis.

PHARMACOLOGY

The same drugs as mentioned above are used. As time goes by more women have a hysterectomy and so then only oestrogens need be taken by these women.

Complications of hormone replacement therapy

MALIGNANCY

There is no evidence of any increase in malignancy of the *cervix* or *ovary*.

Neoplasia of the *endometrium* may follow unopposed oestrogen; the risk increases with the duration of use:

- ×3 to 6 after five years of use.
- ×10 after ten years.

Adding cyclical progestogens virtually eliminates this risk.

Breast cancer is stimulated by higher oestrogen levels. Meta-analysis will indicate relative risk of *breast cancers* is about ×1.1 up to ten years and it is likely to exceed ×1.3 with longer-term therapy. Obviously, a woman with a family history of breast cancer should not be offered HRT because of the increased risk.

CONTINUED PERIODS

The risk rates of cancer of the ovary and cervix are unaffected. Regular monthly bleeding going on into the 60s is a nuisance. It often reduces in amount but still occurs. In attempt to prevent this, progestogens may be given in a wider spread but lower dose throughout the cycle.

Tibolone (2.5mg daily) a gonadomimetic, possesses weak oestrogenic, progestational and androgenic properties. It can be used to treat flushes, psychological and libido problems and is not accompanied by regular withdrawal bleeding symptoms though it is not absolute especially if used on women early in the menopause. Some women have a weight gain due to water retention when they start the oestrogens but this can be controlled after a few months. Some woman get a depression like premenstrual tension during the progesterogen phase. Changing the dose of added progestogens will help this too.

UTERINE ENLARGEMENT

Hyperplasia of the uterus may lead to an increase of bleeding. Any pre-existing fibroids may continue in their growth, whereas normally after the menopause growth stops.

PREMATURE MENOPAUSE

For some the supply of primordial oocytes is not enough and a woman runs out in her mid-thirties. FSH levels will rise in order to try to stimulate the ovaries further, so the woman gets hot flushes but her periods stop.

The diagnosis is confirmed by high FSH levels, combined with low oestradiol concentrations; the tests should be repeated on two occasions. A laparoscopy shows smooth billiard ball-like ovaries. Biopsy of the surface will confirm the absence of oocytes but this is not necessary in most cases when the diagnosis can be more in the under 40-year-old or the biochemical investigations only.

THE CAUSE

This is usually a natural phenomenon due to an absence of oocytes. It will also follow surgical removal of the ovaries, or radiological treatment for malignancy.

Cytotoxic drugs may affect ovarian production but not usually interfere so much with the endocrine production of the ovaries. Some chromosomal disorders, such as Turner's syndrome, and auto-immune disease may cause the ovaries to be poor in oöcytes at the beginning of their reproductive life and so fade early.

MANAGEMENT

Each woman must be carefully assessed for there is a strong psychological element bound up in this condition.

In the *history* enquiry is made about:
• late menarche;
• previous thrombo-embolism;
• liver disease;
• hypertension;
• family history of myocardial infarction or family hyperlipidaemia.

Examination should include a check of the patient's height to assess vertebral compression.

Investigations include oestrogen levels, which are low, and FSH levels which are very high. Normal or raised FSH levels exclude the diagnosis of premature menopause. A laparoscopy would show the ovaries lacking follicles. Vaginal ultrasound can show the absence of follicles developing in the ovaries.

TREATMENT

The woman must be reassured and a full explanation of the biological facts given. Psychiatric help may be required if this is pathologically unacceptable.

Unless there is contra-indication, HRT should be used as discussed already. If the woman does not wish to take hormones or if they are contra-indicated, Clonidine hydrochloride will control vasomotor symptoms and may be helpful. Tranquillizers and antidepressants may be required for insomnia and depression. Pyridoxine (vitamin B_6) is helpful for some.

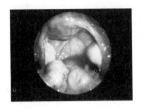

Sexually transmitted diseases

Chlamydia, 144

Gonorrhoea, 144

Syphilis, 146

Human immuno-deficiency
virus infection, 147

Granuloma inguinae, 149

Lymphogranuloma
venerum, 150

Chancroid, 150

It is important that students have knowledge of these diseases, the most widespread infectious diseases in the UK and many other parts of the world.

The increased reported incidence of sexually transmitted disease is due not only to a more liberal attitude to sexual intercourse in most of Western society, but also to the efficiency of clinics in their statistical returns; a statutory requirement in the UK (Fig. 11.1). Sexually transmitted diseases are usually seen in special primary care out-patient clinics for Genito-Urinary Medicine (GUM), formerly known as Venereal Disease (VD) clinics.

As well as the medicine available, at these special clinics there is an efficient service for contacting the sexual partners of those who attend. Obviously there is little point in treating one half of the couple as somebody obviously gave the attender the disease; further there may be an innocent partner who is at high risk of acquiring it. The expert contact tracers and counsellors at the special clinics are an essential part of the treatment of these conditions. Successful therapy eventually depends on reducing the total pool of disease in the community. A gynaecologist should make use of this service if he or she sees a patient with such a condition in the gynaecological clinic.

The two classic venereal diseases were syphilis and gonorrhoea. The former has been largely controlled but the latter is still a common condition. In the last decade, a large number of other conditions which have been shown to be sexually transmitted have been added to the list. The net could be spread wider if we were also to consider certain cancers that are probably sexually transmitted, e.g., cancer of the cervix.

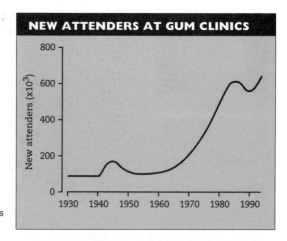

Fig. 11.1 New attendances at GUM clinics.

CHLAMYDIA

Chlamydia is one of the most commonly isolated organisms amongst people attending GUM clinics.

SYMPTOMS AND SIGNS

These are very variable. Commonly there is a vaginal discharge which may be watery or muco-purulent from secondary infection. The cervix is grossly reddened often with an infected erosion.

INVESTIGATIONS

- Chlamydia is difficult to grow and requires a special culture medium.
- Fluorescent monoclonal antibodies can be detected on a vaginal smear with a commercially available kit.
- Enzyme linked immuno-assay is available in most microbiological laboratories.

TREATMENT

- Tetracycline—500 mg four times a day for seven days

or

- Doxycycline—100 mg twice a day for 10 days.

The characteristics of Gardnerella, Trichomonas and Monilia are considered in Chapter 4.

GONORRHOEA

This very infectious disease is spread sexually by Gram negative diplococci which rapidly become intracellular. Numbers of new cases have been reducing for 20 years (Fig. 11.2).

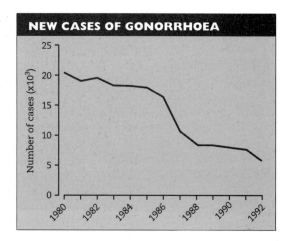

Fig. 11.2 New cases of women with gonorrhoea at GUM clinics 1980–92.

SYMPTOMS AND SIGNS

The gonococcus classically infests the cervix, urethra and Bartholin's glands.

- *Cervix*: recurrent vaginal discharge occurs. It is offensive and yellow-white.
- *Urethra*: urethritis leads to dysuria, particularly at the opening of the urethra on the beginning of micturition.
- *Bartholin's glands*: these become inflamed, occasionally on one side only; this may lead to abscess formation.
- Ascending infection leads to *salpingitis* which can be followed by *infertility*.

INVESTIGATIONS

If the infection is clinically likely, swabs should be taken from the endocervix, the exits of the Bartholin's glands and the urethra after milking some discharge down. The gonococcus is a heat sensitive organism and so either the swabs must be spread straight away on warm blood Agar plates or they should be put into Stuart's transport medium and taken immediately to the laboratory for culture.

It is important to get sensitivity tests because many gonococci are sensitive to standard antibiotics.

Tests for syphilis should be done at the same time, as the treatment of gonorrhoea may mask the symptoms of syphilis without removing all the spirochaetes.

TREATMENT

Most gonorrhoea responds to:
- penicillin—4 million units in 2 doses.

If the organism is resistant to penicillin:

- ampicillin

or

- cephalosporin

or

- Spectinomycin—4g.

If the upper genital tract is involved, as it is in about a fifth of patients, treatment should be continued for several days until the symptoms disappear. Commonly other organisms colonize the vagina and cervix alongside the gonococcus, needing extra treatment. A good example is a trichomonas infection which calls for metronidazole, as anaerobes will have become established with the main infection.

SYPHILIS

This used to be the major sexually transmitted disease but is now comparatively rare. In part this is due to successful treatment of *Treponema pallidum* with antibiotics: furthermore the latent interval is long enough for contact tracing to take place.

SYMPTOMS AND SIGNS

A small papule can occur some weeks after infection on the labia (minor or major) or the fourchette. This is usually pain free and after about 10 days breaks down to an indurated ulcer with a characteristic rolled edge, a chancre, which typically does not bleed.

If left the chancre heals in a few weeks with little fibrosis, leaving enlargement of isolated lymph nodes in the inguinal regions.

Secondary syphilis comes on some months later with a skin rash and general mucosal ulceration. Tertiary syphilis has the classical cardiovascular and neurological symptoms.

INVESTIGATIONS

The papule or chancre is swabbed and the exudate smeared onto a slide. Microscopy with dark field examination shows the presence of spirochaetes.

In secondary syphilis, the serological tests are helpful, but not in the primary phase. These tests are complex but in essence consist of VDRL (Venereal Disease Research Laboratory) and RPR (Rapid Plasma Reagin). These are not specific to syphilis but detect the presence of antibodies. The diagnosis can then be confirmed by FTA (Fluorescent Treponeal Antibody Absorption Test) or TPI (Treponaema Immobilization Test). These are specific and give a true diagnosis of syphilis. The Wasserman Reaction (WR) is no longer used as a specific test.

TREATMENT

- Penicillin – 2–4 million units as two doses intramuscularly; repeat one week later.

If resistant to penicillin:

- tetracycline – 500 mg, four times a day for 15 days.

Follow-up should be at three, six and twelve months. The immunological tests may stay positive much longer than the infection is present.

HUMAN IMMUNO-DEFICIENCY VIRUS INFECTION

Acquired immuno-deficiency syndrome (AIDS) is caused by a retrovirus; in our species that is the human immuno-deficiency virus (HIV). It can insert itself into the host DNA and so is reproduced whenever the cell multiplies. Infection can lead to:

- asymptomatic carriage (HIV carrier);
- AIDS;
- AIDS related diseases.

The presence of antibodies merely shows body response and is not necessarily fully protective.

Transmission occurs through infected body fluids being in contact with the excellular body fluids of the recipient. Thus, semen containing HIV would not cause infection of a women if the epithelium of the vagina or cervix is intact. If, however, there are breaks in the surface such as an erosion of the cervix or a small split of the fourchette, HIV can be transmitted at normal intercourse. Similarly, splits in the anal mucosa at rectal intercourse allow infection at anal intercourse in either men or women. Blood transfusion or the use of blood products can transfer the disease directly from infected donor to the recipient's blood.

The other major route of transmission is the sharing of needles between addicts who are using intravenous injections of illicit drugs. Needles may have been infected by one person and then are often used unsterilized by a second person or more.

Infection must be by direct inoculation into tissues. HIV does not pass an intact skin so does not spread by touching or kissing.

Most women are infected by blood transfusion, receiving blood products or from intravenous drug abuse. In the UK, less than half are infected by their sexual partners who have been infected sexually by others, but in Africa, coitus is the commonest means of transmission of HIV. Males commonly transmit HIV at anal intercourse, probably via minute fissures in the anus sphincter (Fig. 11.3).

The fetus can be infected *in utero* from the mother. About a third of the babies of affected women remain HIV positive at fifteen months;

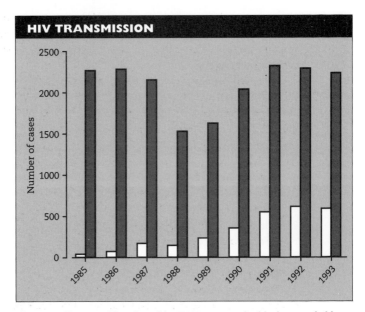

Fig. 11.3 All cases of females with HIV ■ compared with those probably acquired by heterosexual intercourse □.

many of those who were seropositive in the neonatal period were merely reflecting the mother's immunological state.

Transmission may also occur through breastmilk and so in Western countries breast feeding is not recommended although in Central Africa, the epicentre of the HIV, a balance must be made between this risk and that of gastroenteritis from imperfect bottle feeding.

SYMPTOMS AND SIGNS

The full blown picture of AIDS is of recurrent infections in many parts of the body associated with poor resistance to other viral and bacterial infections. The skin and lungs are particularly affected. In the extreme, Kaposi's sarcomata of the skin develop. There are often non-specific symptoms such as prolonged fatigue or weight loss, prolonged diarrhoea, a persistent cough or swollen glands in the neck and axillae.

INVESTIGATIONS

The detection of antibodies in the serum implies contact with either present or past infection; it does not show the current status of the disease.

There are many emotional and financial implications to be considered in the counselling of those who are to be tested for HIV. These must be considered very carefully and the ramifications explored prospectively. Considerations like these curb HIV screening programmes of large numbers, such as those who attend antenatal clinics, because there are not enough professionals available to do adequate prospective screening.

TREATMENT

There is no treatment for AIDS at present. One can only offer supportive therapy, but in future there may be treatment.

- Blocking the entry of the virus to the cell:
    (a) vaccine;
    (b) receptor blocker.
- Blocking replication of the virus:
    (a) DNA polymerase inhibitors;
    (b) block viral protein synthesis.
- Improving the immune cell function:
    (a) bone marrow transplant;
    (b) lymphokine.
    The best treatment at the moment is preventative.
- Screening donor blood for transfusion and blood products.
- Providing clean sterile needles for drug addicts.
- The correct use of condoms at *any* act of intercourse with someone not in regular long-term continuous contact; this applies to homo- and heterosexual contacts.

It is also most important that preventative treatment is employed by all professionals who are in contact with women who have HIV infection or AIDS. Examinations of such women, the taking of blood or cervical smears and operating, demand extra precautions so that the professional is not contaminated with any material. All body fluids produced by such women should be processed separately as should any dressings or swabs, which are associated with body fluids.

The campaign that Governments are mounting to prevent the spread of AIDS by sexual routes must be backed up by a campaign from professionals to prevent the smaller but potentially equally hazardous spread of HIV at the handling of body fluids by attendants of women with the disease. Such precautions should not mask or cover up the empathy which exists in other doctor/patient contacts. Those with HIV need sympathy, not ostracism.

GRANULOMA INGUINAE

This sexually transmitted condition is found mostly in the tropics.

SYMPTOMS AND SIGNS

A painless lump at the vulva breaks down to an ulcer which extends fairly rapidly, thus differentiating it from syphilis. Inguinal glands are involved early, often leading to abscesses in the groins.

INVESTIGATIONS

At examination of the exudate microscopically, Klebsiella-like intra-cellular bacteria are found.

TREATMENT

- Tetracycline—500 mg four times a day for three weeks.

LYMPHOGRANULOMA VENERUM

SYMPTOMS AND SIGNS

A small papule appears on the vulva which later turns into a painless ulcer. Lymph nodes are greatly involved in this condition; they become adherent and to the overlying skin often producing sinuses. Lymphatic blockage follows, leading to elephantiasis of the vulva. The rectum and anal canal may be infected and later stenosed.

INVESTIGATIONS

A chlamydial-like organism can be found in the discharge. Serological tests of immunoflourescence are useful.

TREATMENT

- Tetracycline—500 mg four times a day for three weeks

or

- Sulphamethoxazole—1 g four times a day for three weeks.

CHANCROID

A small painful swelling appears in the vulva which leads on to a painful ulcer. The lymph nodes are enlarged and painful. Only a few lymph nodes are involved in this but often suppurate.

INVESTIGATION

A haemophilus-like organism is found in exudate scraped from the affected tissue.

TREATMENT

- Sulphamethoxazole—1 g four times a day for three weeks.

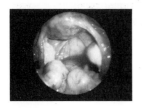

Endometriosis

Definition, 151
  Pathology, 151
  Sites, 152

Diagnosis, 153
Treatment, 157

Hormone therapy, 157
Surgery, 158

DEFINITION

Endometriosis is the existence of endometrium outside the lining of the uterine cavity. This tissue responds to the oestrogen and progesterone variations in the cycle like the normally sited endometrium and, therefore, produces symptoms.

Endometriosis is a disease of women in the second half of their reproductive life, between 30 and 45, and tends to regress at the menopause or even before. The greatest incidence is in women who are childless or have few children; full-term pregnancy leads to regression of the growth, though abortion does not. Endometriosis appears commonest in women of European stock.

Pathology

Deposits of endometriosis consist of endometrial glands and stroma. The tissue bleeds in response to hormone cyclical changes, but there is no escape for the blood, which becomes encysted in areas; infiltration of surrounding structures such as bowel occurs with subsequent fibrosis. These endometriotic areas vary in size from a pinhead to a large cyst with tarry material; the chocolate cyst. Perforation and leakage from tarry cysts in the ovaries leads to dense adhesions to surrounding tissues.

The cause of endometriosis is not known, but there are some important hypotheses on the subject.

• Retrograde spread of collections of endometrial cells shed at menstruation from the uterus, passing along the fallopian tube to the peritoneal cavity. This would account for the highest incidence of endometriosis occurring in the pelvis.

• Blood or lymph borne embolization.

• Metaplasia of the coelomic epithelium.

• Altered immunological recognition of endometrial tissue in some women allowing acceptance of emboli of endometrium in these.

Probably a combination of the first and last theories are the most likely.

Sites

Endometriosis is generally commonest in the pelvis and lower abdomen. It is very occasionally found in bizarre sites such as the pleura, diaphragm, arm, leg or kidney, but these cases are too rare to be part of the practical discussion of the condition.

OVARIES

The ovaries are a very common site for the disease which may take the form of:
• numerous endometrial cysts containing blood;
• a large chocolate or tarry cyst, densely adherent to the surrounding tissues.

Histological examination does not always reveal the presence of typical endometrial glands as these may have been destroyed in large cysts. Cysts larger than 10 to 12 cm in diameter are unusual.

PELVIC PERITONEUM

The pelvic peritoneum is very often affected over the back of the uterus, the fallopian tubes and the pouch of Douglas. Peritoneal deposits, probably secondary to ovarian endometriosis, often present as widespread black nodules with scarring and puckering of the peritoneal surface. Adhesions may form between these, the ovaries and the back of the uterus, causing the uterus to become fixed in a retroverted position.

UTERINE LIGAMENTS

The utero-sacral ligaments and the recto-vaginal septum are often involved. Deposits may be found in the posterior fornix, each appearing as a dense shiny black spot like a pheasant's eye. Endometriosis in the round ligament may be found inside the abdominal cavity or may present as a tumour in the groin if the inguinal end of the ligament is involved.

BOWEL

The intestines and rectum may all become infiltrated with endometriosis. The commonest result is that fibrosis in the wall of the bowel leads to stricture formation and thus to obstruction. Bleeding into the bowel lumen is uncommon.

URINARY TRACT

Endometriosis may occur in the bladder leading to haematuria and painful micturition. Fibrosis around the uterus can follow longstanding endometriosis leading to obstruction of renal flow.

ABDOMINAL WALL

Endometriosis may occur as an isolated lesion at the umbilicus and lead to cyclical bleeding; probably by travelling up a patent urachus. It occurs in scars following operations on the uterus or tubes, particularly those where the cavity of the uterus is opened, such as myomectomy or hysterotomy.

PERINEUM AND VAGINA

Deposits of endometriosis may be seen in perineal scars and in the vaginal wall, though this is uncommon.

Classification

Endometriosis is classified into stages to allow comparison between clusters and grade response to treatment (Table 12.1 and Fig. 12.1).

DIAGNOSIS

This depends on the history, examination and investigations of the patient.

SYMPTOMS

The symptoms of pelvic endometriosis depend on the sites and the activity of the disease. The most typical symptoms occur with endometriosis of the ovaries.

- *Pain*—three main types of pain are found:
  (a) *dysmenorrhoea*, the congestive type, begins before menstruation and is relieved when the flow is established. It is felt in the pelvis and lower back;
  (b) *ovulation* pain is sometimes severe in mid-cycle;
  (c) *dyspareunia* is felt deep in the pelvis due to pressure on the ovaries and recto-vaginal septum during coitus.
- *Infertility* may be the main complaint. This may be due to:
  (a) inability of the ovaries to ovulate;
  (b) ovulation occurring into closed off areas of fibrosis;
  (c) damage to tubal fimbria;
  (d) kinking of tubes by adhesions;
  (e) blockage of tube by deposits of endometriosis in the wall.

STAGES OF ENDOMETRIOSIS

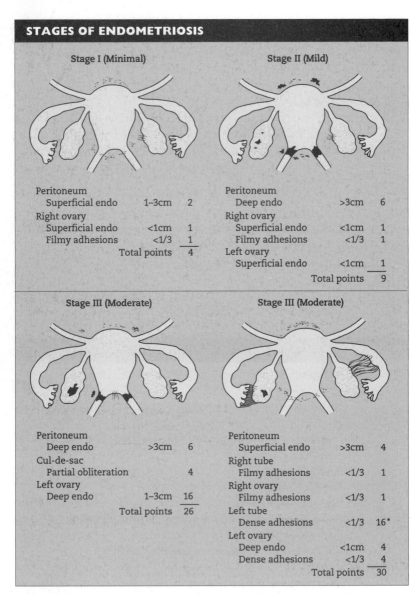

Stage I (Minimal)

Peritoneum
Superficial endo   1–3cm   2
Right ovary
Superficial endo   <1cm   1
Filmy adhesions   <1/3   1
                   Total points   4

Stage II (Mild)

Peritoneum
Deep endo   >3cm   6
Right ovary
Superficial endo   <1cm   1
Filmy adhesions   <1/3   1
Left ovary
Superficial endo   <1cm   1
                   Total points   9

Stage III (Moderate)

Peritoneum
Deep endo   >3cm   6
Cul-de-sac
Partial obliteration   4
Left ovary
Deep endo   1–3cm   16
                   Total points   26

Stage III (Moderate)

Peritoneum
Superficial endo   >3cm   4
Right tube
Filmy adhesions   <1/3   1
Right ovary
Filmy adhesions   <1/3   1
Left tube
Dense adhesions   <1/3   16*
Left ovary
Deep endo   <1cm   4
Dense adhesions   <1/3   4
                   Total points   30

Fig. 12.1 From The American Fertility Society. Revised American Fertility Society Classification of Endometriosis 1985. *Fertil Steril* 1985; **43**:351–2.

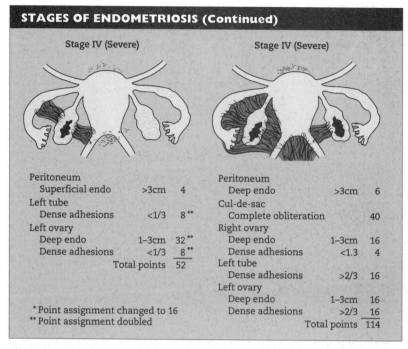

STAGES OF ENDOMETRIOSIS (Continued)

Stage IV (Severe)

Peritoneum		
Superficial endo	>3cm	4
Left tube		
Dense adhesions	<1/3	8 **
Left ovary		
Deep endo	1–3cm	32 **
Dense adhesions	<1/3	8 **
	Total points	52

* Point assignment changed to 16
** Point assignment doubled

Stage IV (Severe)

Peritoneum		
Deep endo	>3cm	6
Cul-de-sac		
Complete obliteration		40
Right ovary		
Deep endo	1–3cm	16
Dense adhesions	<1.3	4
Left tube		
Dense adhesions	>2/3	16
Left ovary		
Deep endo	1–3cm	16
Dense adhesions	>2/3	16
	Total points	114

Fig. 12.1 *Continued*

- *Disturbances of menstruation.* Menorrhagia is a frequent symptom. Short cycles and episodes of prolonged bleeding may occur.

  Other symptoms from endometriosis may be:
- haematuria;
- dysuria;
- intestinal obstruction;
- pain on defaecation;
- occasionally a chocolate cyst may rupture, causing symptoms and signs of an acute abdomen.

PHYSICAL SIGNS

The most typical clinical picture is that of fixed retroversion of the uterus with enlarged, tender ovaries adherent behind it. Deposits in the pelvis may be palpable as tender nodules. Laparoscopy is essential to establish the diagnosis. Many cases are not diagnosed until laparotomy.

DIFFERENTIAL DIAGNOSIS

- *Chronic pelvic infection* most closely resembles pelvic endometriosis, the

CLASSIFICATION OF ENDOMETRIOSIS

Size of deposits	< 1 cm	1–3 cm	> 3 cm
Peritoneum			
Superficial	1	2	4
Deep	2	4	6
Ovary			
Right superficial	1	2	4
Deep	4	16	20
Left superficial	1	2	4
Deep	4	16	20
Adhesions			
Ovary			
Right film	1	2	4
Dense	4	8	16
Left film	1	2	4
Dense	4	8	16
Tube			
Right film	1	2	4
Dense	4	8	16
Left film	1	2	4
Dense	4	8	16
Pouch of Douglas			
Partly obliterated	4→		
Completely obliterated	40→		
Score			
1–5 Minimal			
6–15 Mild			
16–40 Moderate			
>40 Severe			

Table 12.1 Classification of endometriosis from The American Fertility Society. Reproduced with permission of the publisher.

symptoms of premenstrual dysmenorrhoea, menorrhagia, sterility and dyspareunia being identical, but the history and laparoscopy findings being different.

• *Fibroids* of the uterus are often associated with endometriosis, but the differential diagnosis of both may be difficult.

- *Carcinoma of the ovary* with multiple metastases in the pelvic peritoneum can present clinically in a similar way to endometriosis.

TREATMENT

Treatment of pelvic endometriosis is essentially conservative because the condition:
- tends to occur during the later reproductive period;
- does not become malignant;
- tends to regress at the menopause.

Hormone therapy

This is successful in many cases. The diagnosis must first be made at laparoscopy and if there are large chocolate cysts these must be removed; local areas of endometriosis can be coagulated with laser through the laparoscope.

Danazol inhibits pituitary gonadotrophin secretion and in adequate doses will suppress menstruation. The initial dose is 400 mg daily in divided doses, increasing up to 800 mg daily. Treatment should be given initially for six months. There may be mild androgenic effects:
- acne;
- hirsutes;
- weight gain due to fluid retention.

It is important to be sure that the woman is not pregnant and it must be stressed that Danazol is not a contraceptive.

Progesterone used to be the major therapy, using norethisterone starting on the fifth day of menstruation with 10 mg daily and increasing up to 40 mg daily. Nausea, vomiting, weight gain and fluid retention may occur.

An alternate progestogen is medroxyprogesterone acetate (10 to 30 mg daily by mouth). The object is to suppress menstruation for six months. If break through bleeding is troublesome, an oestrogen such as ethinyl oestradiol 0.05 mg daily for 21 days out of 28 may be given.

Side effects are common with both hormone treatments, but in patients who persist regression of the endometriotic lesions occurs and pregnancy may become possible, though ovulation may be delayed for several months after treatment.

Synthetic substitutes of *gonadotrophin releasing hormone* (GnRH) and their agonists are inhibitors of ovarian function. Two weeks treatment (subcutaneously or nasal spray) reduces FSH and LH concentrations and leads to lower oestrogen levels. Treatment for three to six months gives relief. Side effects may be:

- headaches;
- hot flushes;
- depression;
- loss of bone density if treatment long enough.

Surgery

Very small lesions may be treated by diathermy or laser through the laparoscope. Laparotomy is indicated in:

- pelvic masses over 5 cm;
- acute rupture of a cyst;
- intestinal obstruction.

Conservative surgery is always performed if possible, aiming to leave some normal ovarian tissue. All areas of endometriosis are excised or cauterized.

In intractable cases, and especially among women who do not want children, wider surgery may be needed. Hysterectomy may be performed for intractable menorrhagia and dysmenorrhoea or when there are fibroids or adenomyosis. Some ovarian tissue may be left if not actually involved in the destructive process.

CHAPTER 13

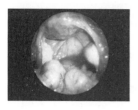

Prolapse of the genital tract

Retroversion of the uterus, 159

Causes, 159
Prolapse, 162

Classification, 162
Treatment, 166

In the standing adult woman, the uterus is in the centre of the true pelvis; in the majority, it is anteverted—the fundus directed forwards, and anteflexed—the body of the uterus bent forward on the cervix (Fig. 13.1).

However, vaginal examinations take place with the woman lying down. Then the body of the uterus often angles back to become axial, i.e., in line with the long axis of the vagina. Hence, while it is true that in the anatomical position four-fifths of uteruses are anteverted and one-fifth retroverted, at vaginal examination, about 40% are anteverted, 40% axial and 20% retroverted (Fig. 13.2).

The structures which maintain the position of the uterus are:
- the cardinal or transverse ligaments;
- the utero-sacral ligaments.

These are attached to the sides of the supravaginal cervix and lower uterus, leaving the body of the uterus mobile in all directions and capable of growth during pregnancy. The normal uterus is mobile, altering its position when the bladder or rectum become distended. The secondary support of the uterus is the muscular pelvic floor.

RETROVERSION OF THE UTERUS

The fundus of the uterus is directed backwards; this is usually accompanied by backward flexion so that the uterus is:
- retroverted;
- retroflexed.

Causes

In many, retroversion is the normal position. There may be a shallow

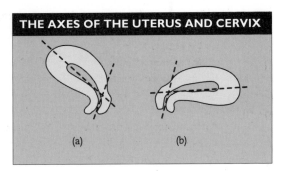

Fig. 13.1 The relation of the axes of the uterus and cervix. (a) Anteverted, antiflexed. (b) Retroverted, retroflexed.

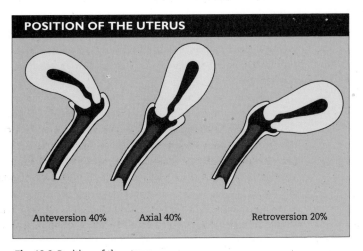

Fig. 13.2 Position of the uterus.

anterior vaginal fornix; the congenitally retroverted uterus tends to revert to this position after childbirth.

Acquired retroversion results from four main groups of causes.

• In *puerperal* retroversion, the heavy recently pregnant uterus falls backwards into the pouch of Douglas after delivery. Spontaneous return to the anteverted position usually occurs.

• *Prolapse* retroversion of the uterus often occurs when the organ becomes prolapsed on account of the weakening of its supports. Retroversion is also commonly seen in the *senile uterus* even without prolapse; the tiny uterine body falls backwards.

• *Fixation by adhesions* may tether the body of the uterus in the retroverted position. Adhesions commonly result from salpingitis, endometriosis and malignant disease, especially carcinoma of the ovary.

- *Displacement by a tumour.* Tumours which may displace the uterus backwards include:
    (a) uterine fibroids;
    (b) an ovarian tumour;
    (c) distended bladder.

SYMPTOMS

An uncomplicated retroversion of the uterus causes no symptoms. The decision may have to be made whether to inform a woman about a retroverted uterus. If she is told, the importance of it must be played down, especially in a woman who is already introspective about her pelvis.

Possible symptoms may be:
- dyspareunia;
- menorrhagia;
- infertility;
- recurrent abortion;
- backache.

DIAGNOSIS

The diagnosis of retroversion of the uterus is made on bimanual examination and depends on the following three points:
- the cervix points forward;
- the body of the uterus is felt through the posterior fornix in the pouch of Douglas;
- the body of the uterus is not felt by the abdominal hand. Examination should be made with the bladder, and preferably the rectum, empty.

TREATMENT

No treatment is required in retroversion causing no symptoms and discovered in routine examination. Operative correction of retroversion for functional symptoms such as spasmodic dysmenorrhoea or menorrhagia is very likely to give disappointing results.

Pessary treatment may be used if retroversion appears to be responsible for infertility or habitual abortion. A specially moulded pessary is a rigid plastic Hodge pessary (Fig. 13.3). It is important to replace the uterus into the anteverted position before inserting the pessary and this may not be easy. Insert one or two fingers into the posterior vaginal fornix and displace the body of the uterus upwards out of the pouch of Douglas. With the other hand above the pubes, the fundus is now scooped forward while the fingers in the vagina displace the cervix backwards.

The pessary is now inserted and should fit snugly and comfortably between the posterior vaginal fornix and the anterior vaginal wall, above

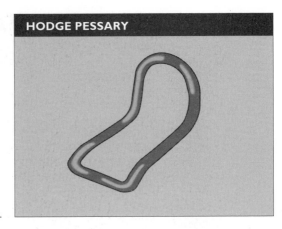

Fig. 13.3 A Hodge pessary.

the urethral orifice (Fig. 13.4). The pessary is left in position for three months and then removed to see if the uterus falls back again and, if so, if the symptoms recur.

The operative treatment is ventrosuspension by:
- intraperitoneal shortening of the round ligaments;
- Gilliam's operation, drawing a loop of the round ligament on each side lateral to the rectus muscle and suturing it to the inner surface of the anterior rectus sheath.

PROLAPSE

Prolapse is a downward descent of the female pelvic organs due to weakness of the structures which normally retain them in position. Both descent and prolapse are relative terms and perceived differently, but are more frequently encountered in women who have borne children and rarely in nulliparous women. Prolapse does not usually become apparent until after the menopause when there is general shrinking and weakening of the supports of the pelvic organs. It is less common in Black races.

A prolapse resembles a hernia for there is protrusion of part of the abdominal contents through an aperture in the supporting structures. Protrusion takes place between the two levatores ani and, in more severe cases, through the orifice of the vagina.

Classification

Six components of genital prolapse (Fig. 13.5) are recognized.

HODGE PESSARY IN PLACE

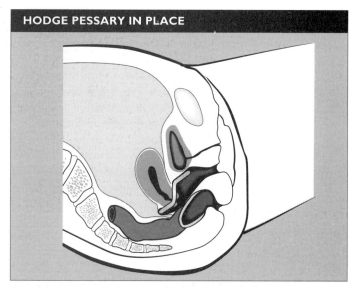

Fig. 13.4 A Hodge pessary in place comfortably.

GENITAL PROLAPSE

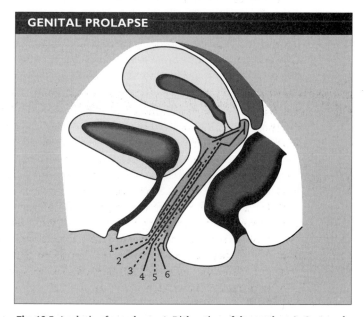

Fig. 13.5 Analysis of a prolapse. 1. Dislocation of the urethra. 2. Cystocoele. 3. Descent of cervix and uterus. 4. Enterocoele. 5. Rectocoele. 6. Deficient perineum.

1 *Dislocation of the urethra* is a condition in which the urethra is displaced downwards and backwards off the pubis. It may be also dilated becoming an urethrocoele. This arises from damage to or weakness of the triangular ligament.

2 *Cystocoele* is a hernia of the bladder trigone following weakness of the vaginal and pubo-cervical fascia. The bladder base descends and later a bladder pouch is formed which may contain residual urine.

3 *Uterine prolapse* is descent of the uterus and cervix.

(a) *First degree* with a descent of the uterus, but the cervix remains within the upper vagina.

(b) *Second degree* uterine descent, when the cervix reaches down to the vulva on straining, but does not pass through it.

(c) *Third degree* or *procidentia* when the cervix and some or all of the uterus is prolapsed outside the vaginal orifice. In practice the fundus of the uterus usually remains within the vagina, but there is an associated inversion of the vagina. The outer covering of the prolapse consists of the completely inverted vaginal wall and it contains the uterus, the bladder and utero-vesical pouch, the considerably elongated pouch of Douglas and part of the rectum.

4 *Enterocoele* or pouch of Douglas hernia is a prolapse of the upper part of the posterior vaginal wall. The hernia contains the peritoneum of the pouch of Douglas often with a loop of bowel. Enterocoele may occur concurrently with other types of genital prolapse, especially procidentia. It is also seen in prolapse following abdominal or vaginal hysterectomy.

5 *Rectocoele* is a prolapse of the lower part of the posterior vaginal wall due to weakness or divarication of the levatores ani; the rectum bulges into the vagina.

6 In posterior wall prolapse, *the perineal body* may be deficient and part of the anal canal may bulge into the vagina. Deficient perineum often results from inadequately sutured tears after childbirth or by failure of union of such tears.

SYMPTOMS

Symptoms of genital prolapse are variable and do not bear much relation to the physical signs found on examination. They probably relate to the degree of traction on the pelvic ligaments. The symptoms tend to progress with the day's activities and can be relieved by lying down. Below the commonest complaints are listed.

- A feeling of fullness of the vagina.
- A lump coming down.
- A dragging sensation or bearing down in the back or lower abdomen.
- Vaginal discharge due to congestion of the cervix, an infected tear, an

ulcer of the ectocervix or cervical erosion. A bloodstained discharge may occur if there is ulceration.

• Difficulty with coitus may be experienced if the cervix protrudes or is greatly elongated.

• Urinary symptoms may be:

(a) *frequency* of micturition is common and is often diurnal only;

(b) *nocturnal frequency* may be present if there is added cystitis;

(c) *urgency* of micturition due to weakness of the bladder sphincter mechanism and urge incontinence may occur in some cases;

(d) there may be *difficulty in emptying* the bladder completely and the woman may find she has to push the prolapse up with a finger before she can complete the act of micturition;

(e) complete *retention of urine* is seen due to overstretch of the urethra;

(f) *stress incontinence* when mild is common in women even without prolapse. This is considered in Chapter 14.

• Rectal symptoms:

many women with prolapse complain of constipation and this may be due to difficulty in emptying the rectum completely because it bulges into the vagina. Others notice discomfort on sitting on a firm surface; the vaginal wall over the rectocoele can bulge down between the labia. With age, the labia becomes atrophic and less protective and the prolapsed vagina is exposed to trauma when sitting on hard surfaces.

PHYSICAL SIGNS

The woman should first be examined in the dorsal position when she is asked to strain and cough. While she does, the anus may be supported to spare her the embarrassment of an involuntary escape of flatus or faeces. In case of doubt, she may be asked to stand up or walk about for a short time before testing for prolapse again on the bed.

The degree of descent of the cervix is tested with a finger in the vagina.

Where there is a complaint of stress incontinence, examination is best made with some urine in the bladder; the urethra and bladder neck may then be supported with two fingers to demonstrate that this manoeuvre controls the incontinence.

DIFFERENTIAL DIAGNOSIS

The diagnosis of prolapse is not difficult; it may be difficult to decide if it is the cause of the patient's main symptoms. Prolapse must be distinguished from:

- vaginal or periurethral cysts;
- tumours of the cervix or vagina;
- a diverticulum of the urethra;
- urethral caruncle;
- urethral mucosal prolapse.
  Symptoms similar to those of prolapse may be caused by:
- varicose veins of the vulva;
- haemorrhoids;
- rectal prolapse;
- cystitis;
- vaginitis with congestion of the vagina;
- backache;
- pressure from a large abdominal tumour.

Stress incontinence must be distinguished from other causes of incontinence of urine such as urge incontinence and incontinence due to neurological disease. Senile incontinence occurs in very old women without stress. A fistula between the bladder, urethra or ureter and the vagina may be present. Such a fistula may be minute and careful investigation may be necessary.

PREVENTION

Careful management of labour is important. The woman must be discouraged from bearing down before full dilatation for this may damage the uterine supports. The second stage of labour should not be prolonged unduly; episiotomy and low forceps extraction may reduce the risk of vaginal prolapse. Episiotomies and tears must be carefully sutured in layers. Postnatal exercises should be encouraged after every labour. All women should see a physiotherapist to help with this.

Prevention of vault prolapse after hysterectomy is helped by suture of the cardinal and utero-sacral ligaments to the vaginal vault. Subtotal hysterectomy is more likely to lead to vault prolapse than total hysterectomy, even though many women ask for the former.

Treatment

Treatment of prolapse may be palliative or operative.

PALLIATIVE TREATMENT

Many types of pessary and support have been devised for prolapse. Their use is only temporary, the better cure being a repair operation. With modern techniques of surgery and anaesthesia, operation can safely be undertaken in the majority of cases of prolapse.

The indications for pessaries are:

- prolapse during pregnancy;
- prolapse immediately after delivery;
- when another pregnancy is desired within a short time;
- in patients unfit for operation on medical grounds;
- in patients who refuse operation.

PESSARY TREATMENT

A plastic ring pessary which fits well surrounds the cervix, pointing slightly forward, and resting between the posterior fornix and the anterior vaginal wall (Fig. 13.6). It supports a vault prolapse by stretching the vaginal wall while a cystocoele is directly supported by it. It is less successful in controlling a rectocoele; if the perineum is grossly deficient, the pessary will tend to slip or even fall out.

Pessaries are made in 5 mm sizes from 50 to 120 mm.

There are a few cases where a ring pessary fails to control prolapse and operation cannot be performed. In these cases there are other appliances. The cup and stem pessary consists of a sheet of vulcanite or plastic with a stem to which are attached tapes which are tied to a belt. It is removed at night for cleaning and is thus less likely to cause ulceration. It is a useful long-term pelvic floor support.

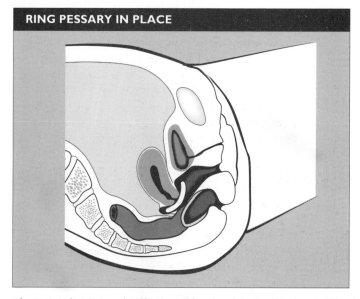

RING PESSARY IN PLACE

Fig. 13.6 A ring pessary in place stretching the vaginal wall and so holding up the uterus.

Disadvantages
- Ulceration of the vagina and cervix.
- A neglected pessary may become embedded in the vaginal wall and may only be removed with great difficulty.
- A carcinoma of the vagina may develop.

PHYSIOTHERAPY

This has a limited place, chiefly in young women after recent childbirth where the vaginal walls and pelvic floor are mainly affected. It is less effective in vault prolapse. Exercises to strengthen the pelvic floor muscles are carried out under the supervision of a physiotherapist including the voluntary retention of weighted cones in the vagina to strengthen the pelvic muscles (Fig. 13.7). This may be combined with faradism to the pelvic floor muscles.

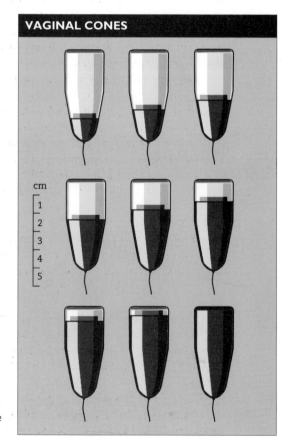

VAGINAL CONES

Fig. 13.7 A set of vaginal cones to help pelvic floor exercises improve muscle tone.

SURGERY

The best operation for repair depends on the degree of descent of the various components of the genital tract together with the judgement and expertise of the surgeon.

Anterior colporrhaphy and *posterior colpoperineorrhaphy* may be combined with *amputation of the cervix* and shortening and suture of the cardinal ligaments; this is the Fothergill or Manchester operation.

The reasons for amputating the cervix are:
• the supravaginal cervix may be elongated;
• after suture of the cervix, repair of the vaginal vault is more satisfactory;
• the cervix is often unhealthy and infected;
• a possible site for future carcinoma has been removed.

The cervix will not be amputated in young women who may wish to bear children and in cases where there is no vaginal vault prolapse.

Many surgeons perform *vaginal hysterectomy* when operating for prolapse, an operation of choice when prolapse is combined with menorrhagia or where there are small uterine fibroids. Vaginal hysterectomy may be preferred in cases of uterine procidentia.

Abdominal operations may be combined with prolapse repair, for example ventrosuspension when the uterus is much retroverted. Abdominal hysterectomy may be required for large fibroids and the prolapse may be repaired at the same operation or later. Removal of a large tumour may itself lead to cure or improvement of prolapse.

Stress incontinence presents surgical problems. It can occur with or without prolapse and may be one of the most difficult symptoms in gynaecology to cure. Details of surgical repairs are given in Chapter 14.

PRE-OPERATIVE CARE

Preparation for operation is most important. The general condition of the patient is assessed and treatment given for conditions such as obesity and chronic cough. Cardiovascular disease and mild diabetes are common in middle-aged women and may need preoperative treatment.

Ulceration of the vagina can follow exposure of the vaginal tissues outside the body in a procidentia or from long-wearing of a ring pessary. The pessary should be removed some days before surgery and the patient may need to have rest in bed in hospital with the prolapse reduced.

Urinary tract infection is common and must be treated. Urge incontinence and detrusor muscle instability should be treated with antispasmodics and surgery postponed until this urogynaecology aspect is fully treated.

In postmenopausal women, atrophy of the vagina may delay healing; preoperative treatment may be given with oral oestrogens, pessaries or as dienoestrol cream.

POST-OPERATIVE CARE

Early movements and deep breathing are encouraged and the patient should get out of bed as soon as possible. The use of a lavatory or commode in private helps to overcome difficulties with micturition and defaecation. Laxatives are given as required.

There can be post-operative complications in the first two weeks after gynaecological operations.

- *Chest complications* associated with general anaesthesia.
- *Retention of urine* and urinary tract infection. Retention usually requires catheterization. If extensive dissection, especially of the perineal tissues, is carried out during the operation, an indwelling catheter should be inserted at the operation. There are the two types: a urethral Foley catheter or suprapubic Bonano catheter. The bladder should be drained continuously for three to five days and the catheter then clamped intermittently for a day to reintroduce the sensation of bladder filling. An antibiotic agent should be given during continuous catheterization to prevent urinary infection.
- *Local sepsis* is frequent; rarely there is spread of infection with pelvic peritonitis or parametritis.
- *Haemorrhage* may be primary, reactionary or secondary. Blood transfusion may be required and in secondary or reactionary haemorrhage, resuturing of the vagina or cervix to arrest bleeding and packing of the vagina will be required under anaesthesia in the operating theatre.
- *Pelvic vein thrombosis* and *pulmonary embolism* may occur.
- *Adhesions* may form in the vagina and should be gently broken down with the gloved finger about five days after operation at a postoperative vaginal examination check.

There are remote complications.

- *Vaginal discharge* may persist for some weeks. In some cases it is due to granulation tissue in the scars; this may be treated with silver nitrate. Sutures used in the repair may not be absorbed. They can be nicked and any excess suture material removed at two weeks.
- *Urinary complications* include frequency due to irritable bladder or chronic infection. Stress incontinence may persist in spite of careful surgery. Rarely a vesico-vaginal or urethro-vaginal fistula develops.
- *Dyspareunia* is common and may be caused by leaving the vagina too small; care must be taken not to reduce the vaginal circumference, especially if a posterior repair follows an anterior wall operation. Dyspareunia may also result from disuse of the vagina due to fear. Senile

atrophy may also be seen in the age group of those having repair operations.

PROGNOSIS OF FUTURE PREGNANCIES AFTER PROLAPSE REPAIR

Successful pregnancy can be achieved after prolapse repair though if the cervix has been amputated there may be an increased tendency to miscarry. Caesarean section is advisable in most cases especially if there is fibrosis of the remaining cervix, if there has been an extensive vault repair or where operation has been done for severe stress incontinence.

Vaginal delivery may be allowed in some cases; deep episiotomy should be performed and the perineum carefully repaired in layers.

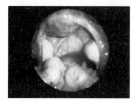

Urogynaecology

Physiology, 173
Urinary incontinence, 174
　Urinary fistula, 174
　Genuine stress
　　incontinence, 174
　Detrusor instability, 175
Overflow incontinence,
　175
Reflex incontinence, 176
Urodynamic investigation
　of incontinence, 176
Treatment, 177
　Stress incontinence, 177
The unstable bladder,
　178
Overflow incontinence,
　179
Urinary tract infection, 180
Urinary frequency, 180
Nocturnal enuresis, 181

PHYSIOLOGY

The bladder has two main functions.
- To act as a reservoir for the storage of urine.
- To empty this reservoir away from the skin of the body at an appropriate time and appropriate place.

Acting as a reservoir, the bladder:
- is lined with waterproof transitional epithelium which does not allow diffusion of the urinary constituents across its wall;
- is a sac with high compliance. It can accommodate a large volume of urine (300 to 500 ml) with very little rise of intravesical pressure (0 to 15 cm H_2O);
- is able to expand suprapubically and extraperitoneally without hindrance or constraint by bone or pelvic viscera;
- maintains the pressure in its outflow tract along the urethra at a higher level than intravesical pressure thus preventing leakage of urine.

The bladder is an efficient expulsive organ.
- The smooth detrusor muscle is richly innervated by the parasympathetic nervous system outflow of sacral roots 2, 3 and 4.
- At the onset of micturition the pelvic floor striated muscle is voluntarily relaxed, reducing the intraurethral pressure. The background inhibition of the sacral reflex arc is suppressed. Efferent impulses pass to the detrusor muscle causing a rise in intravesical pressure. This then exceeds the intraurethral pressure and leads to the passage of urine down the urethra.

URINARY INCONTINENCE

The involuntary loss of urine may be due to:
- urinary fistula;
- genuine stress incontinence;
- detrusor instability (urge incontinence);
- overflow incontinence;
- reflex incontinence.

Urinary fistula

A pathological tract may open between a part of the urinary system and an epithelial surface such as that of the vagina or occasionally the skin. These tracts bypass the normal controlling mechanisms causing development of continuous (true) incontinence. They can be congenital or follow major radical surgery or disease such as cancer of the cervix.

• Congenital (rare); draining the upper pole of one kidney and opening into the anterior wall of the vagina. They present in children with continuous urinary loss. Result in poorly functioning renal polar hydronephrosis and an ectopic hydro-ureter.

• Caused by major radical surgery—avascular necrosis leads to weakening of the wall of the ureter or bladder and the development of a ureteric or vesico-vaginal fistula.

(a) Gynaecological surgery, particularly if there has been anatomical distortion by infection, endometriosis, carcinoma or by preceding small blood vessel damage (endarteris) caused by irradiation.

(b) Obstetric trauma, particularly in association with obstructed labour where the presenting part causes avascular necrosis of the bladder base or sometimes the rectum, causing the development of a vesico-vaginal and recto-vaginal fistula respectively.

Genuine stress incontinence

An involuntary loss of urine occurs from the urethra, when the transmitted intra-abdominal pressure causes a rise of the intra-vesical pressure which exceeds the intra-urethral pressure in the absence of a detrusor contraction. Approximately 25% of older women have mild problems and 5 to 10% severe.

SYMPTOMS

Involuntary urine loss associated with a sudden, usually unexpected, rise of abdominal pressure such as coughing, sneezing, laughing or lifting.

PHYSICAL SIGNS

The coincidental downswing of the bladder neck with urinary leakage from the urethra with the legs apart in the standing and often lying positions.

About 50% are associated with prolapse of the vagina.

Detrusor instability

Incidence—8 to 10% increasing with age.

AETIOLOGY

Incompletely understood but may be due to:

• an abnormality in the central nervous system when anxiety and stress result in the loss of ability to inhibit at the detrusor reflex and, therefore, the development of detrusor contraction;

• associated with a recognized neurological defect, such as spinal trauma, demyelinating disorders or epilepsy;

• may be associated with intense bladder inflammation, particularly in the elderly.

SYMPTOMS

• Urgency of micturition leading to urgency incontinence—an inability to hold on.

• Frequency of micturition both by day and night.

• May also be associated with stress incontinence.

DIAGNOSIS

The demonstration of detrusor contraction (more than 15 cm water) on cystometry, provoked by bladder filling or straining and the movement or sound of running water.

Overflow incontinence

Loss of urine when the bladder has become overfilled, usually associated with either:

• obstructive surgery to the bladder neck;

• denervation of the detrusor muscle (usually by extensive pelvic surgery).

SYMPTOMS

• The frequent passage of small volumes of urine.

• Hesitation of micturition.

- A slow stream.
- A sensation of incomplete emptying.
- Involuntary leakage when bending down or getting up out of a chair.

PHYSICAL SIGNS

- A palpable bladder.
- Leakage on elevation of bladder base.
- On cystometry, slow urine flow rate.
- High residual urine.
- Risk of back pressure to upper urinary tract if chronic.

Reflex incontinence

Reflex involuntary voiding associated with sensory stimulation of the sacral 2, 3 and 4 segments. This develops when the higher centres are cut off from the sacral reflex arc and thus micturition ceases to be centrally suppressed. It is triggered when there is a significant increase of the afferent impulses to the sacral segments 2, 3 and 4 either from the bladder or the somatic nerves.

Detrusor contractions are often associated with a simultaneous contraction of the pelvic floor (detrusor dysynergia) causing partial obstruction of urine flow, unlike the relaxation in centrally organized normal micturition.

URODYNAMIC INVESTIGATION OF INCONTINENCE

- Bladder behaviour can be assessed by keeping fluid output charts to measure the frequency of the volumes of urine passed during the day.
- Cystometry (with subtracted abdominal pressure) determines the presence or absence of involuntary detrusor contractions thereby differentiating the stable from the unstable bladder and these pressure measurements may be coupled with video radiological screening (Figs 14.1 and 14.2).
- The residual urine can be measured by catheter or pelvic ultrasound.
- Measurement of urinary flow rate with pressure measurements differentiates the obstructed urethra from the poorly functioning detrusor.
- Ultrasound urograms outline defects of the bladder and upper urinary tract and retrograde urography to demonstrate ureteric and vesico-vaginal fistulae.

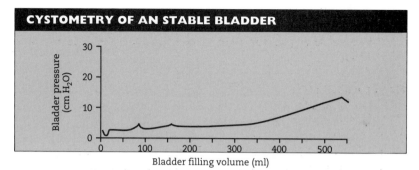

Fig. 14.1 Cystometry of a normal bladder filling with rise in intravesical pressure.

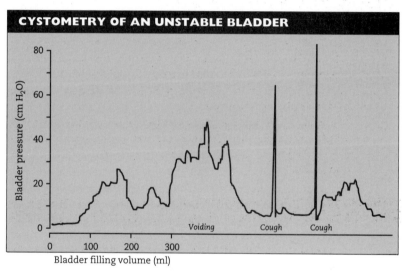

Fig. 14.2 Cystometry of filling an unstable bladder.

TREATMENT

Stress incontinence

Conservative
• Mild urinary leakage (particularly postnatally)—with a good physiotherapist and patient motivation, pelvic floor exercises usually result in improvement.

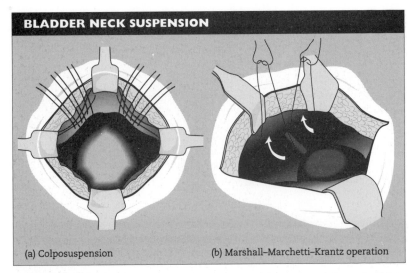

BLADDER NECK SUSPENSION

(a) Colposuspension   (b) Marshall–Marchetti–Krantz operation

Fig. 14.3 Bladder neck suspension operations. Each aims to resuspend the neck of the bladder to the periosteum of the pubis (a) or the iliopectineal ligament (b).

- Reduction of weight, excessive physical exertion and the treatment of coughing also helps.

Surgical
- Vaginal approach—anterior colporrhaphy with bladder neck buttress is a simple operation and permits repair of other prolapses at the same time. Long-term success rate in curing incontinence is approximately 40%.
- Sling operation—multiple varieties—using synthetic substances (nylon, prolene, Teflon, mersilene mesh) or natural tissues (e.g., round ligament or external oblique aponeurosis). Insertion is by open surgery or blind by directed needles through the retropubic space (e.g., Stamey procedure).
- Retropubic bladder neck suspension operations—suturing the vaginal wall to the pectineal ligament (Burch) or paravaginal tissues to the back of the pubic symphysis (Marshall–Marchetti–Krantz) (Fig. 14.3). These procedures are associated with an 85 to 90% cure rate of the incontinence but do not remedy much prolapse apart from that of the anterior vaginal wall.
- Para-urethral infection of collagens to stimulate fibrin formation.

The unstable bladder

There is often a psychosomatic element (Fig. 14.4). The symptoms are improved by several means.

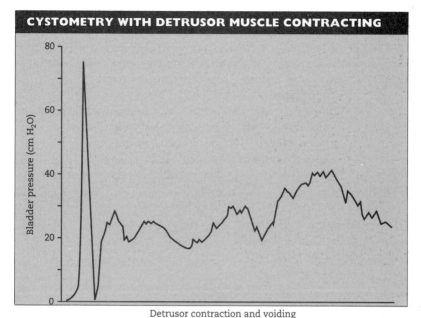

CYSTOMETRY WITH DETRUSOR MUSCLE CONTRACTING

Detrusor contraction and voiding

Fig. 14.4 Cystometry with detrusor muscle contraction and voiding.

- Enthusiastic encouragement, with the help of urinary output volume chart, particularly by incontinence advisors, district nurses and doctors. If necessary admission to hospital for intensive bladder training under close supervision.
- The use of anticholinergic drugs, e.g., oxybutynin, probanthine, imipramine.
- The use of vaginal oestrogen cream to reduce bladder irritability and the tendency of recurrent urinary infection.

Overflow incontinence

- If obstructed, the urethral dilatation or urethrotomy results in improvement.
- If due to weakened detrusor muscle—continuous drainage with a suprapubic catheter for two to three weeks to improve the tone of the detrusor often helps with subsequent bladder training. Occasionally intermittent self-catheterization can be of assistance although infection is common.

URINARY TRACT INFECTION

Almost all urinary tract infections develop by the upward spread of the bacteria along the 5 cm of urethra. Infections are associated with:
- the upward massage of organisms during intercourse;
- catheterization;
- the incomplete emptying of the bladder leading to stagnant urine;
- lack of oestrogens leading to atrophic urethritis;
- poor hygiene following defaecation or intercourse;
- vaginitis and cervicitis.

SYMPTOMS

- Burning dysuria.
- Severe urinary frequency and strangury.
- Urgency of micturition.
- Suprapubic discomfort.
- Urine odour.

    If the infection has spread beyond the bladder to the upper part of the urinary tract then:
- loin pain;
- vomiting;
- rigors.

INVESTIGATIONS

- Dipstick impregnated with nitrate sensitive amine to screen for bacteria.
- Mid-stream urine culture.
- Cervical or high vaginal swab culture.

TREATMENT

- Encouragement of high fluid intake.
- Rest in bed if temperature is raised.
- Rapid use of antibiotics.
- Use of topical oestrogens in postmenopause women.
- Educational hygiene encouraging post coital micturition and correct wiping after defaecation.
- Bladder training with suprapubic catheter if the residual urine volumes are high.

URINARY FREQUENCY

Is associated with:
- bladder irritants, e.g., coffee, cola and fortified wines;

- the presence of calculi;
- high fluid intake resulting in an increased urinary output;
- diabetes mellitus may present with polydypsia and polyuria;
- the use of diuretics;
- anxiety, tension and stress, e.g., outside the examination hall;
- development of habits and rituals at home or at work associated with a particular voiding pattern;
- insomnia leading to nocturia;
- the reduction of peripheral oedema overnight resulting in increased kidney excretion, bladder filling and nocturia.

NOCTURNAL ENURESIS

The involuntary voiding of urine into the bed clothes whilst asleep.

AETIOLOGY

Not fully known, but the following associations have been noted:
- deep sleep leading to the loss of suppression of the voiding reflex;
- impairment of the kidneys to concentrate urine whilst asleep, for example by the persistence of daytime renal excretion pattern;
- psychological disturbances such as great unhappiness;
- bladder instability in later life.

TREATMENT

- Frequent waking overnight to ensure regular voiding.
- The use of desmopressin and nasal sprays to suppress urine formation whilst asleep.
- Mattress alarms.
- Imipramine.

CHAPTER 15

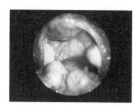

Sexual problems

History and examination, 183

The male, 184
  Failure to ejaculate, 184
  Premature ejaculation, 185

Erectile dysfunction, 186

The female, 187
  Superficial dyspareunia, 187
  Deep dyspareunia, 188
  Vaginismus, 188

Anorgasmia, 189

Rape, 190

Criminal abortion, 190

Annulment of marriage, 191

Many students do not like considering patients' sexual problems, for they feel they have hardly sorted out their own sexual lives let alone being in a position to help others. A more open discussion of this subject helps the student to be at ease when discussing sexuality later with patients. It helps the students to become more aware of their attitudes and how these may influence the future doctor/patient relationship.

Patients often consult their doctors about sexual problems and expect them to have the knowledge and skills to help them. Following the increase in public awareness of sexuality will come a higher rate of consultation. Further, it is necessary for a doctor to know the interrelation of sexually related matters and their treatments to general diseases such as heart disease and hypertension.

The facts of human sexuality have not been always known but by proper analysis, assessment and randomized controlled trials of various therapies, more is becoming comprehensible.

HISTORY AND EXAMINATION

As with the rest of medicine, a schematic approach to sexual problems can help make a diagnosis. A full general and gynaecological history should be taken including details of past gynaecological events, the type of contraception used and obstetrical history.

The sexual problem should be discussed allowing the woman or man to use their own phrases, preferably in their own time. If they wander, pointed questions drawn from the following material may be needed to bring them back to the point.

QUESTIONS

- Duration and frequency of intercourse.
- Factors improving.
- Factors making problem worse.
- Happens with other partners.
- Other associated factors such as alcohol, work or drugs.
- Other life events at the time of onset.
- The relationship of the partners.
- History of previous sex knowledge.
- Family background to sex education in childhood.
- Past sexual relationships.
- Present sexual history.
- Details of usual sex activities—e.g., position and foreplay.
- Sexual fantasies.
- What improves or worsens the sexual relationship.
  Examination is usually unrewarding.
- In the male—obvious abnormalities of the penis and testes should be excluded.
- In the female—the ease of allowing a pelvic examination may be helpful in assessing the degree of the problem. Any structural abnormalities of the vulva, vagina, cervix or uterus should be excluded. The examination can be used positively as an opportunity to educate about genital anatomy. The use of a mirror to help a woman identify her clitoris can be helpful.

It is important to detect general physical abnormalities which might make intercourse difficult or painful before exploring the possibility of psychosexual problems. The patient's comfort or discomfort with their own body and specifically genitalia can give useful information.

THE MALE

Although this is not strictly a part of gynaecology, anyone dealing with sexual problems must have knowledge of the male partner and his problems.

Failure to ejaculate

The inability to produce semen is not always associated with the sex drive itself or the ability to have an erection.

CAUSES

- Sympathectomy.
- Psychosexual features:

(a) past humiliating sexual rejection;
(b) fear of a pregnancy in partner;
(c) past maternal domination;
(d) repressive sexual teaching as a child;
(e) doubts about sexual orientation.

TREATMENT

Sympathectomy aspects can be treated with drugs.
* Thioridazine
or
* Indoramin.

The psychological aspects may require long-term psychotherapy, because many cases are due to the man avoiding depositing semen in his partner's vagina; this produces further anxieties.

Lesser degrees can be dealt with by sympathetic handling by the woman and extra-vaginal sexual techniques. The encouragement of the use of erotic material can help if there is loss of control at the point of ejaculation.

Premature ejaculation

Ejaculation occurs with minimal stimulation or before or shortly after penetration and before either party wishes it.

Ejaculation is under sympathetic control mediated by adreno-receptors. It probably means that the mediated system enhances this whilst the serotonin balance is inhibitory. These equilibria may be over-ridden by behavioural patterns.

CAUSES

Behavioural patterns are associated with:
* inexperience;
* adolescent conditioning to rapid response;
* rejection by other women.

TREATMENT

Men can be treated individually or with their partners. Sympathetic handling by the woman is important. Male confidence must be generated as he learns to recognize the point of ejaculatory inevitability and to control stimulation to delay ejaculation until the time of his choosing. A squeeze technique applied by the woman to the penis at the moment before ejaculatory inevitability can produce delay in ejaculation. If a programme is embarked on over the course of weeks or months, this produces good results.

Drugs are occasionally helpful if there is poor response to the psychological approach:
• Clomipramine
or
• 5HT reuptake inhibitors may be helpful.

Erectile dysfunction

Impotence in the male may be primary or secondary. The former is nearly always psychological due to problems in the family background/ upbringing while secondary impotence may be physical or psychological.

CAUSES

Structural
• After major pelvic operations.
• Pudendal vein thrombosis.
• Hypospadias.
• Peyronie's disease (fibrosis of the dorsum of the penis).

Endocrine disease
• Diabetes.
• Hypogonadism.
• Hypothyroidism.
• Pituitary tumour.
• Cushing's syndrome.

Medical problems
• Peripheral vascular disease.
• Hypertension.
• Cerebral vascular accident.
• Multiple sclerosis.
• Spinal cord injury.
• Increasing age.

Drugs which can be associated
• Alcohol.
• Antihypertensives.
• Antidepressants.
• Antipsychotics.
• Hormones.

Psychological features
• Stress.

- Performance pressure.
- Parental influence.
- Ignorance of sexual matters.
- Poor self image.
- Guilt.
- Anger.
- Relationship problems.

It is important to differentiate the psychogenic from the organic causes. The former are associated with:

- rapid onset;
- a recent depression;
- life or family stress;
- normal erections:
    - (a) on waking;
    - (b) masturbation;
    - (c) in response to erotic material;
    - (d) with a different partner.

TREATMENT

Psychological treatment starts with reassurance and education leading on to non-demand, touching exercises based on Masters and Johnson's sensate focus programme.

Erection can be produced by pharmacological means.

- Papaverine injected into the corpus cavernosum works by smooth muscle relaxation.
- Other injectable drugs are phentolamine and prostaglandin E_1. These work particularly for men with spinal cord injuries.
- Yohombine by mouth may assist dysfunctional male erection.
- Some of the drugs used for the treatment of medical conditions such as hypertension may be changed for others with less effect on the erectile function.

THE FEMALE

Superficial dyspareunia

Vaginal pain during intercourse may be due to a variety of causes. Physical causes of superficial dyspareunia include:

- infection of the vulva or vagina;
- dermatological disease of the vulva or vagina;

- postmenopausal atrophy;
- painful perineal scar from episiotomy;
- an undilated hymen—this is very rare and mostly related to women who maintain virginity into the late 30s.

TREATMENT

Dealt with according to the cause. Surgical reconstruction may be required for badly healed episiotomy or a rigid undilated hymen.

Deep dyspareunia

This is felt higher up in the vagina and in the pelvis. It often lasts for some hours after intercourse and can be reproduced at vaginal examination by pressing over relevant parts of the female pelvis.

CAUSES

- Chronic pelvic infection.
- Endometriosis.
- Pelvic tumours including unruptured tubal ectopic pregnancy.
- Adhesions or uterine retroversion trapping ovaries in the pouch of Douglas.
- Pelvic congestion.
- Bladder or bowel pathology.
- Failure of arousal response. Superficially this is due to failure of lubrication and deeply due to failure of vaginal ballooning during coitus.

TREATMENT

That of the basic cause; results depend on the responsiveness to the treatment of physical problems.

Results where no pathology is demonstrated are variable. In these women, dyspareunia may be due to intra- or inter-personal conflicts. The use of lubricants and delay of penetration until the woman is fully aroused can be helpful.

Vaginismus

Spasm of the superficial and deep pelvic muscles prevent the introduction of the penis and is apparent at a pelvic examination.

CAUSES

There may be an organic cause but usually it is a psychological result of apprehension and fear. Previous attempts at forced entry may lead to this.

TREATMENT

A sympathetic approach to examination can help, but no force should be used. Attempts should stop before pain is caused and the woman should feel in control at all times.

Occasionally examination under anaesthesia may be required to exclude structural causes and thus be able to reassure the woman that she is anatomically normal. Usually this is not necessary as she is likely to respond to gradual desensitization techniques. To this end, the use of graduated vaginal trainers is often helpful. Fingers or tampons are sometimes preferred. Referral to a trained sex therapist may be needed.

Anorgasmia

This is not uncommon in the female. This is nearly always psychological, but in a small percentage it is physical. About 10% of women remain anorgasmic.

CAUSES

A failure to:
- receive stimulation — psychological in origin;
- respond to stimulation — due to family upbringing/background;
- performance pressure from partner or self;
- doubts about sexual orientation.
  Other causes:
- fear of pregnancy;
- dyspareunia;
- debilitating disease;
- chronic constipation.

TREATMENT

Mechanical and organic causes are treated appropriately. Psychological causes require the attention of a sex therapist who would discuss the problem fully with the individual or the couple.

Too easily the woman is labelled as frigid and then accepts this as a part of life. Fifty per cent of women are not orgasmic during penetrative sex, but are orgasmic with clitoral stimulation. Understanding this can help remove pressure from both partners to achieve coital orgasm on every occasion.

Treatment usually involves helping the woman to achieve orgasm through masturbation and learning to lose control. The use of erotic material or a vibrator can help. Progress to coital orgasm is then made. Use of vibrators may also help with coital orgasmic problems.

RAPE

Rape is unlawful sexual intercourse with a woman against her will; only the slightest penetration of the vulva by the penis is required. Issues of whether the hymen is intact or if semen has been deposited in the vagina are irrelevant.

Rape is unfortunately all too common and the woman may report it to the police, sometimes a day or so later. A doctor may then be called to examine the victim of alleged rape. The practitioner should ensure that he or she has the authority and consent for the examination and has the equipment for taking the appropriate specimens properly.

A history of what happened is taken and careful notes made. Examination is made of the general demeanour of the woman and of her clothing. Bruises and scratches around the lower abdomen, thighs and vulva should be noted, preferably in a diagrammatic form. The vulva should be examined in detail for bruising or tears.

If any suspicion of semen in the vagina is found, a careful specimen should be taken, placed in appropriate containers and labelled fully in the presence of a woman police constable (WPC) and the complainant. This should then be handed to the WPC for examination in forensic laboratories and a receipt received.

Other swabs and blood may be taken to exclude sexually transmitted diseases. While these often have no legal standing, they may be important in the medical management of the woman's future.

Many police forces have a rape investigation team who are able to satisfy both the law and the psychological needs of the woman who is in this situation. A knowledge of the procedures involved is still helpful to all practitioners.

CRIMINAL ABORTION

One of the results of the laws about therapeutic termination of pregnancy in England, Wales and Scotland, has been the massive reduction in criminal abortions. Not a single death has been reported in the last nine years covered by the Confidential Enquiries into Maternal Deaths (1982–1991). This is a very satisfactory situation in the UK but criminal abortion still goes on throughout the world. It is estimated that of the half a million women who die every year of maternity causes, about a quarter do so from incompetently performed non-legal abortions.

If a doctor is asked to examine a woman who may have undergone a criminal abortion, he or she first must obtain her consent if she is conscious.

HISTORY

This should be taken but may be only partly truthful.

EXAMINATION

The woman may be pyrexial and ill with dull pain in the lower abdomen. Pelvic examination may show the cervix to be soft and the os dilated. Blood or pregnancy tissue may be passing through it. There may be signs of the bite of a volsellum (toothed forceps) on the anterior lip of the cervix. She may have an offensive discharge coming through the cervix. Damage to the genital tract may occur, e.g., the posterior fornix is commonly perforated by incompetent abortionists who force their instruments into the cul-de-sac of the vagina and penetrate it, breaching the peritoneal cavity.

TREATMENT

The woman should be admitted to hospital. Antibiotics should be given urgently, a broad spectrum used at first until the results of high vaginal swabs are known. Consider the diagnosis of gas gangrene and if relevant give anti-gas gangrene serum. If the woman is still bleeding from the uterus, a curettage may remove septic products from the cavity and hasten healing. Check the haemoglobin level; a blood transfusion may be required for toxic anaemia. Watch for anuria which commonly follows gross toxic infection.

Whilst confidentiality to the patient is the first concern of the doctor, if the woman becomes seriously ill or approaches death, legal authorities may be involved. Take advice about this from the legal department of the hospital or the doctor's defence society or union. Keep careful notes.

ANNULMENT OF MARRIAGE

In certain circumstances a marriage can be dissolved by divorce on the grounds of non-consummation. In the case of a woman, an Inspector of Nullity appointed by the Courts may be expected to examine her to certify if the woman has not had normal sexual intercourse. Alternatively, the Inspector may have to attest that there is no impediment to the consummation of marriage or that if one is present it could be cured. The task of the Inspector in respect of nullity in the case of the male partner is rather more difficult to describe or fulfill.

This ground of divorce is not used so often now but there are still some 80 gynaecologists appointed Inspectors of Nullity to the Courts in England and Wales.

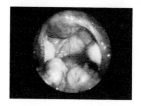

Infertility

Causes of infertility, 193
Investigation of the
   infertile couple, 194
   History from the female,
      194
   Examination of the
      female, 195
   History from the male,
      195
   Examination of the male,
      195
   Investigations, 195

Treatment of infertility,
   199
   Correction of coital
      difficulties, 200
   Measures to improve
      cervical secretions, 200
   Sperm hostility, 200
   Lesions of the uterine
      body, 200
   Lesions of the tubes, 200
Treatment of male
   infertility, 202
   Phase one, 203

Phase two, 203
Assisted fertilization, 204
   Gamete intra-fallopian
      tube transfer (GIFT),
      205
   Other methods, 205
   Zygote intra-fallopian
      transfer (ZIFT), 206
   In utero injection (IUI), 206
   Direct injection of sperm
      into oocyte, 206
   Artificial insemination,
      206

Infertility is present when pregnancy does not occur after one year with unprotected coitus at frequent intervals, approximately two or three times a week.

CAUSES OF INFERTILITY

BOTH PARTNERS

- Mechanical difficulty in coitus with inadequate penetration, often associated with lack of ability in the male to maintain an erection.
- Periods of separation so that there is no intercourse at the most fertile time.

MALE

- Impotence.
- Premature ejaculation.
- Azoospermia.
- Deficiency in the sperm count.

FEMALE

- Intact hymen—a woman may complain of sterility when her marriage has not been consummated.

CAUSES OF ANOVULATION
Primary ovarian dysfunction
Genetic e.g., Turner's syndrome Autoimmune
Secondary ovarian dysfunction
Disorders of gonadotrophin regulation
Hyperprolactinaemia
Functional
Weight loss
Exercise
Gonadotrophin deficiency
Pituitary tumour
Pituitary infarction
Pituitary ablation
Polycystic ovary syndrome

Table 16.1 Causes of anovulation.

- Vagina—congenital malformation.
- Uterus—congenital malformation, or tuberculous endometritis.
- Fallopian tubes—infection may close or partly obstruct.
- Ovaries:
    (a) ovulation may not occur;
    (b) ovulation is irregular with anovulatory cycles (Table 16.1);
    (c) polycystic ovarian disease;
    (d) Short luteal phase cycle;
    (e) Anovular cycle—endometriosis, ageing ovary.
- General diseases:
    (a) obesity;
    (b) thyroid deficiency;
    (c) diabetes;
    (d) chronic nephritis.
- The most important factors are:
    (a) male—poor performance and deficient sperm count;
    (b) female—deficient ovulation and blocked fallopian tubes.

INVESTIGATION OF THE INFERTILE COUPLE

History from the female

Age, occupation, length of time with partner, use of contraception or avoidance of pregnancy, previous sexual activity.

Previous pregnancies, including abortions, induced or spontaneous.

Menstrual history; age at onset, cycle and duration of flow, dysmenorrhoea, ovulation pain, recent change in the cycle.

Vaginal discharge; character, amount, whether associated with irritation or soreness.

Previous illnesses, especially tuberculosis.

Operations, especially in the abdomen or pelvis.

Coitus-frequency, difficulties, relation to fertile days.

Previous investigation or treatment of infertility.

Examination of the female

- General examination—physical development, evidence of endocrine disorder.
- Abdominal examination—scars, tenderness, guarding, masses.
- Vaginal examination—state of introitus, position and direction of cervix, position, size and mobility of the uterus, uterine enlargement, enlargement or thickening of the tubes or ovaries.
- Examination with a speculum—conditions of cervix, cervical secretion in relation to time in menstrual cycle.

History from the male

- Age, occupation, including absence from home, length of time with partner and duration of infertility.
- Sexual performance—frequency, ability to ejaculate in upper vagina.
- Previous relationships, fathering of any pregnancies.
- History of mumps with orchitis, injury to genitalia or operations for hernia or varicocoele, any recent debilitating illness.

Examination of the male

- General build and appearance.
- Examination of genitalia, hypospadias.
- Palpation of testicles, size, consistency. Relate size to standard models (Fig. 16.1).

Investigations

POST COITAL TEST

This is done within a day or so of expected ovulation. The couple are advised to have intercourse 12 hours before the test; the woman should

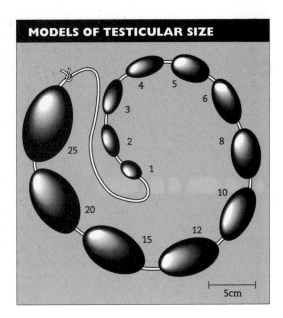

MODELS OF TESTICULAR SIZE

5cm

Fig. 16.1 Models of testicular size to allow a standardization of the examined testes size with an objective comparison.

not bath or douche. Cervical mucus is aspirated under direct vision from the cervical canal and is examined under the microscope for the presence of more than five actively progressive motile sperms per high power field.

Absence of sperms may mean deficiency in the male, mechanical difficulty in coitus or non-receptive cervical secretions. Immotile sperms may indicate that the test is being performed too long after intercourse or is not being performed at the time of intercourse. Sperm antibodies in the cervical mucous may cause immobility.

The presence of leucocytes may indicate inflammation of the prostate or seminal vesicles or cervical infection.

SEMINAL ANALYSIS

Best performed on a masturbation specimen which should be examined within two hours of collection. It should not be from semen ejaculated at intercourse using a condom as most modern sheaths are lubricated with spermicidal cream.

The motility of sperms is important—direct, straight moving sperms being the more likely to effect fertilization.

There should be at least 20 million sperms per millilitre with a total count of not less than 100 million. Fertility reduces progressively with numbers below this. Abnormal forms should not exceed 40%. Reliance should not be placed on a single sperm count.

NORMAL SEMINAL ANALYSIS

Volume	2 to 5 ml
Liquifaction time	Within 30 minutes
Count	20 to 150 million/ml
Motility	> 40% motility at 1.5 hours
Sperm morphology	> 60% normal forms

Box 16.1 Expected values at a normal seminal analysis.

In cases of azoospermia the cause should be sought. It may be due to primary hypogonadism, when the level of gonadotrophic hormone will be high, or the secondary hypogonadism where gonadotrophic hormone will be low; in the latter case there may be excess of prolactin secretion, usually due to a pituitary tumour and possibly responsive to bromocriptine. Other causes of azoospermia may be related to congenital absence of the vasa deferentia or to obstruction in the epididymis.

SPERM ANTIBODIES

The cervical mucus contact test may be used to confirm sperm antibodies; clear cervical mucus and spermatozoa from the couple are mixed on a slide and examined under a microscope. In cases of sperm hostility the sperms show no progression, but a shaking phenomenon or an agglutination head-to-head or tail-to-tail.

A crossed hostility test using donor semen and donor cervical mucus as well may indicate if one partner is generating antibodies (Fig. 16.2). Antibodies can be detected early in the peripheral plasma.

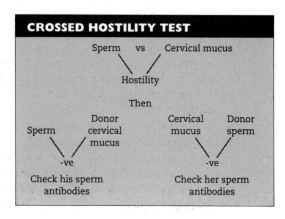

Fig. 16.2 Crossed hostility test.

BASAL TEMPERATURE CHARTS

The woman should keep charts of her basal temperature for a period of three months. This is best taken first thing in the morning before leaving bed. In theory, the raised progesterone levels elevate the basal body temperature by 0.3 to 0.5°C within 12 hours of ovulation. The graphic chart produced bears some relation to ovulation when the ovulation is regular (Fig. 16.3). However, the correlation of temperature to ovulation is less easily seen when ovulation is irregular. Other extraneous causes of temperature fluctuation (e.g., 'flu) intrude on this test as do unusual life rhythms (e.g., nurses on night duty).

EXAMINATION OF THE ENDOMETRIUM

A sample may be obtained by a Vabra endometrial biopsy in the out-patients department or a full curettage. The endometrium should be

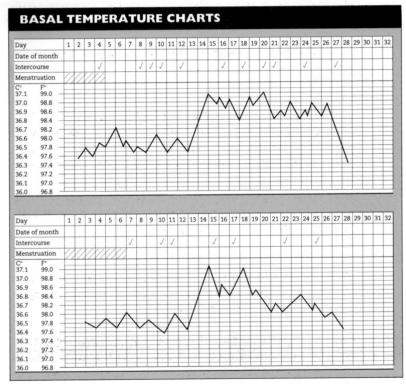

Fig. 16.3 Two basal temperature charts (see text for details). The upper shows a sustained rise of basal temperature from day 12 indicating a pregnancy. The lower chart shows the temperature rise to be unsustained and indicates a fault in implantation and death of the blastocyst.

examined in the premenstrual phase of the cycle. Histological examination will show secretory changes as evidence of ovulation. Tuberculosis is excluded by histological examination and culture.

TESTS FOR TUBAL PATENCY

Tubal patency may be tested under direct vision at laparoscopy. A solution of methylene blue is injected through a tightly fitting cannula in the cervical canal. The passage of the dye may be observed. When the tubes are normally patent the dye pours out of the fimbriated end of the tube into the pouch of Douglas. Tubal obstruction may be recognized as can the presence of adhesions; a hydrosalpinx may be seen to fill with dye which does not spill.

Hysterosalpingography may be done to evaluate blockage of the tubes and to show the site of the obstruction; it can also demonstrate a congenital malformation of the cavity of the uterus which will not be apparent at laparoscopy. A new contrast medium containing microbubbles may be injected transcervically and its passage along the fallopian tube detected with ultrasound.

The carbon dioxide insufflation test for tubal patency is rarely done now because of the dangers of gas embolism.

HORMONE TESTS

Serum progesterone levels in mid second half of cycle (Days 21 to 23 of a 28 day cycle) are two or three times as high as those of the rest of the cycle (15 ng/ml compared with 3 to 6 ng/ml) if ovulation has occurred. If not, FSH rather than LH levels should be checked for they are more specific of ovulation.

Prolactin levels should also be measured to exclude microadenomata of the pituitary gland; levels above 1000 mu/l are significant and should lead to CT scan of the pituitary fossa.

ULTRASOUND

An ultrasound scan of the pelvis, especially with a vaginal probe gives excellent views of the ovaries and uterus if there may be pathology in either (e.g., polycystic ovary syndrome).

TREATMENT OF INFERTILITY

A couple seeking medical advice for infertility are obviously anxious and concerned. They should always be offered help even if the period of infertility is relatively short. A full investigation may take up to six months and it should not be hurried.

About 25 to 30% of women seeking advice for infertility become pregnant during investigation and treatment. There are various lines of treatment which may prove successful depending on the condition found.

Correction of coital difficulties

An intact hymen should be removed or dilated; where there is a tight perineum, perinotomy may be needed. A vaginal septum may have to be removed but usually they cause little difficulty. The woman should be taught to pass vaginal dilators and this helps to give her confidence. The use of a lubricant at coitus also helps.

In the male, the commonest problems with fertility are premature ejaculation and inadequate erection. Both of these are discussed in Chapter 15.

Measures to improve cervical secretions

Where cervical secretion is deficient or unusually viscous, the use of oestrogen in the first ten days of the cycle may improve matters; ethinyl oestradiol 0.01 to 0.02 mg may be given for 10 days beginning on the first day of the period. The dose should not be larger than this or withdrawal bleeding will occur and ovulation may be inhibited. The couple should have intercourse as often as they wish from the 11th to the 15th day.

Infected erosions of the cervix should be treated by electro-cauterization or cryosurgery.

Sperm hostility

Despite apparently normal ovulation and sperm production, sperm antibodies may be demonstrated in one partner. In some cases steroid suppression may be tried.

Lesions of the uterine body

Removal of uterine polypi at curettage is often successful. Myomectomy should be performed if the fibroids are blocking the fallopian tubes or are submucous. Laparoscopy or laparotomy may reveal other conditions such as endometriosis or peritubal adhesions which require relevant therapy.

Lesions of the tubes

Various operations may be undertaken to restore patency and function in cases where the tubes have been damaged by infection.

- *Salpingostomy* where the fimbrial end is opened and held open by turning out a cuff.
- *Tubal reimplantation* where the isthmus is blocked. The medial tubal end is freed and is reimplanted into the uterine cavity.
- *Salpingolysis* where peritubal adhesions are divided.
- *Reanastomosis* if the tube is blocked in mid segment; the obstructed area is resected and the open ends reanastomosed often using microsurgery.

Results of many of these operations are disappointing because:

- *patency* can easily be restored but the tube may be too rigid to allow peristalsis;
- *infection* may have caused the tube to be fixed to other organs by adhesions and so the fimbrial end cannot manoeuvre to the ovary and thus harvest the oocytes;
- after surgery there may be *too short a length of tube* so that the fertilized oocyte passage may be too short and the endometrium might not yet be ready to receive it.

In consequence, the success rates of tuboplasty after infection range from 2 to 10%. The best results come after reanastomosis of sterilization procedures when most surgeons will report a 40 to 60% success rate, which can be improved to about 75% by the use of microsurgery. Despite these poor results there are some women who will be prepared to submit to such an operation even though the hope of a successful pregnancy is slight.

In cases of non-ovulation, further investigation is indicated.

- *Hormone levels* may be estimated in the blood. FSH, LH and oestradiol may be estimated at weekly intervals.
- *Laparoscopy* may reveal atrophic ovaries, multiple small cysts of the ovaries as in the polycystic ovary syndrome or endometriosis. These need appropriate treatment.

Biopsy of the ovary may be performed at laparoscopy.

If there is a high level of prolactin on more than one occasion a CT scan should be done to exclude a pituitary tumour. Excess of prolactin is treated with bromocriptine 2.5 mg daily for three days, then 2.5 mg twice a day for three to six months or longer.

Cases of primary or secondary ovarian failure show high levels of FSH and low levels of oestrogen. Induction of ovulation is probably impossible for there are no more oocytes, but the patient should be given oestrogen replacement therapy if she needs it.

Cases of ovulation failure with low FSH and LH levels may be treated by the use of combined gonadotrophins. Human menopausal gonadotrophin (hMG) contains both gonadotrophins with a higher proportion of FSH and it is the more powerful preparation. hMG is sold as Pergonal, which must be given carefully to prevent hyperstimulation, leading to multiple ovulation and thence to multiple pregnancy.

Giving gonadotrophins should be monitored with oestrogen plasma levels; results must be obtained inside the same working day. The plasma oestrogen levels reflect the action of the gonadotrophins on the ovary. In practice, 150 iu of hMG are given for two days from about day eight of cycle. The dose is increased daily in the first half of the cycle, depending on the oestrogen levels each day and ultrasound examination of the ovary which shows the number and size of follicles coming towards ovulation. When the response is satisfactory, an injection of hCG is given which acts in a similar manner to LH. Once a satisfactory dosage pattern has been established in one cycle, this can be repeated in other cycles in up to six treatment courses or until a pregnancy is achieved.

Occasionally, luteinizing hormone releasing hormone (LHRH) or less specifically pulsatile gonadotrophin releasing hormone (GnRH) is required to stimulate the production of LH from the anterior lobe of the pituitary gland. This must be given intravenously; for the patient who is not in the hospital, this is done most easily with a portable pump worn round the waist or carried on the shoulder, injecting pulses of LHRH into the circulation.

Cases of ovulation failure with low FSH and LH levels but normal oestrogens may be treated with clomiphene citrate; the dose is 50 mg daily for five days commencing on the third day of menstruation; a basal temperature chart should be kept to indicate ovulation or levels may be estimated. Treatment should be repeated provided menstruation occurs and it is certain that the woman is not pregnant. If the first course is unsuccessful, three further courses using 100 mg may daily be used and treatment with 150 mg daily given for the next three cycles. The woman should be examined regularly for hyperstimulation of the ovaries; in general it is unwise to continue for more than six or seven months but some women conceive after treatment is stopped. Clomiphene has also been used in combination with hCG for cases of luteal phase deficiency.

Tamoxifen (Nolvadex), 10 mg twice a day for four days from the second day of the period and Cyclofenil 100 mg twice a day for ten days from the first day of menstruation are both recommended for the treatment of non-ovulation though it has not been shown that they are any better for this purpose than clomiphene.

TREATMENT OF MALE INFERTILITY

If it has been established that male factors are associated with infertility, treatment can proceed. This is best done in two phases:

- less invasive treatments;
- more specific therapies.

Phase one

The first phase should last about three months. Two specimens of semen should be examined to establish levels in the sperm count. Certain aspects of the man's way of life may need to be altered:

- over-exertion;
- excessive smoking;
- excess alcohol consumption;
- poorly controlled diabetes;
- hypertension;
- being overweight.

If the scrotal temperature is raised, it is wise to wear boxer shorts to allow the testes to hang in a cooler atmosphere but older recommendations to hold the scrotum in iced water for varying lengths of time do not help.

The timing of intercourse may need discussion so that at the time of ovulation, the man produces his best semen. A few days of abstinence before this may boost the count if there is a deficiency; otherwise timing is irrelevant.

Any varicocele causing a raised temperature of the scrotum and the efferent ducts from the testes is managed by ligation. Three-quarters of men improve their sperm count after this if the varicocele has been a feature.

Phase two

Specific treatments will depend upon the results of investigations. A low sperm count with low FSH and testosterone level may indicate treatment with stimulating hormones.

In the absence of hormone deficiency, endocrine therapy is less easily justified. However, if the FSH levels are normal clomiphene (25 mg a day for 25 days) has been shown to be of help. Testosterone (200 mg a week for 20 weeks) may temporarily suppress spermatogenesis so that on cessation, there is a rebound increase in sperm levels. Other androgens may also be used in lower therapeutic levels but they are less helpful. Hypoprolactinaemia is rare in most males, but if it is present then bromocriptine should be used.

Impaired fertility is associated sometimes with an increased incidence of chronic prostatitis. If present, long-term, low-dose antibiotic treatment may remove this potential cause (erythromycin 250 mg twice a day for a month).

Sperm antibodies should be checked in the male plasma. If present, they may be treated by immunosuppression with cortisol but it must be stressed this is a treatment with major side-effects especially on the gastrointestinal system and the skeleton. Sperm washing has been described with variable results. Ejaculated sperm is washed in phosphate buffer saline and resuspended for artificial insemination. This aims to wash the antibodies from the surface of the sperm.

Generally speaking, the management of male factors of infertility is disappointing and the success rate usually ranges between 20 and 40%.

ASSISTED FERTILIZATION

Artificial fertilization methods have increased in use greatly in the last decade with probably over 10000 children in the world born as a result. Artificial fertilization has received considerable media cover but should be considered as only one part of infertility management, particularly for those who cannot transmit sperms or eggs along the fallopian tubes due to their damage or absence (Box 16.2).

Patients selected for programmes are usually under 38 years of age and in a stable relationship. They should be free of medical or psychological disease and the woman should have a normal uterus.

TECHNIQUE

For the process to take place, it is essential that oocytes be recovered. Most women now have ovarian cycles stimulated by gonadotrophins for several days before the potential time of ovulation and LH is given to stimulate ovulation. This can be monitored by daily ultrasound scanning when follicle size can be measured; the follicle should measure about 20 mm diameter for oocyte recovery.

Harvesting this may be done through a laparoscope under general anaesthesia. More usually now, the operator aspirates the oocytes through the posterior fornix of the vagina or bladder under local anaesthesia guided by ultrasonic scanning. Usually several (3 to 15) oocytes are recovered at the same procedure.

INDICATIONS FOR *IN VITRO* FERTILIZATION (IVF)

Cause of infertility	%
Disease or absence of the tubes	50 to 70%
Endometriosis	7 to 15%
Sperm abnormalities or low count	5 to 20%
Sperm antibodies	1 to 5%
Idiopathic infertility	3 to 15%
Failed donor insemination (DI)	1 to 5%

Box 16.2 Indications for *in vitro* fertilization (IVF).

The oocytes used to be mixed on a warmed flat dish in special media with semen obtained from the husband by masturbation which has been diluted. Fertilization took place *in vitro* and under specially controlled conditions of temperature and atmospheric gases. The eggs were allowed to develop to the eight cell stage, and were then introduced to the woman's uterus through the cervix, using a fine cannula in as atraumatic a fashion as possible. Up to three fertilized ova were reinserted at the correct time in the cycle.

There may be a place for luteal support with progesterone or hCG in the days following embryo replacement if there has been long exposure to anti-progestogen drugs like buserelin.

RESULTS

Success rates at established IVF units are about 15 to 20% per cycle. Success should be judged by a live birth and not just by the implantation of a fertilized egg—a biochemical pregnancy shown by a rise in hCG levels.

Gamete intra-fallopian tube transfer (GIFT)

If the tubes are present and patent but conventional methods have failed, one may use Gamete Intra-Fallopian tube Transfer (GIFT). The oocytes are recovered at laparoscopy under general anaesthesia. Prepared mobile sperm from the male semen is then passed through the laparoscope into the fallopian tube and one or two of the oocytes are put into the same tube. The whole procedure takes about half an hour and there is no extracorporeal phase. Success rates slightly better than those of IVF are being claimed (30 to 35% per cycle).

Other methods

Increasingly, society is accepting the use of *surrogate parenthood*. If a woman has no uterus or has had it surgically removed, she still can make oocytes. Gametes, fertilized by her partner, can be cultured in the uterus of another woman, perhaps a relative such as a mother or a sister. This baby is genetically from the parents and only lodges for 38 weeks in the body of another.

Other variations include donated oocytes or sperm if such gonodal material is unavailable naturally. The baby is legally the child of the woman who bears him, i.e., the surrogate woman.

Zygote intra-fallopian transfer (ZIFT)

Zygote Intra-Fallopian Transfer (ZIFT) puts fertilized ova back into the fallopian tube two days after fertilization instead of replacement into the uterine cavity as in GIFT.

In utero injection (IUI)

Washed semen are injected into the uterine cavity in the hope of meeting an oocyte by travelling up the tube as happens naturally.

Direct injection of sperm into oocyte

Micromanipulation is performed at special centres placing an individual sperm under the zona and into the oocyte.

Artificial insemination

Artificial insemination by the husband (AIH) or by a donor (AD) may be used in those where impotence or premature ejaculation leads to difficulty. The woman may be taught self insemination using a cervical cap or a syringe. Success rates are 5 to 10% per ovulation.

In some cases where the male is infertile insemination with donor semen (DI) may be considered; this is best done by a doctor. Careful counselling of the couple about the implications is essential. Success rates are 15 to 40% per ovulation.

DONORS

Facilities should be available for accumulating a sperm bank with samples from young donors preferably of proven fertility. A sufficient variety of donors must allow the matching of height, hair colour and race by the doctor in charge of DI.

SAMPLES

Samples are produced by masturbation and are usually divided into tubes or straws of about 0.5 ml each so that the average donor will produce enough to fill six to ten tubes at any ejaculation. These are stored in liquid nitrogen under careful conditions and checked every two years.

DI AND HIV

Until recently, fresh semen was used for DI; this was marginally better at achieving pregnancy than using frozen semen. One of the major fears of artificial insemination has become the theoretical risk of contamination from HIV. In consequence, all donor units now check their donors for HIV antibodies at the time they produce their sample. The samples are then frozen and the donor is rechecked three months later in case he was incubating AIDS at the time he produced the sample. If the second test is negative then the sample can be used for insemination. The percentage of pregnancies achieved is less than with fresh semen by 10 to 20%.

TECHNIQUE

The woman is positioned comfortably and a speculum inserted to expose the cervix. Insemination is usually performed into the cervical canal with recently defrosted semen; not more than 0.5 ml of semen is used because it would be painful to distend the canal with a greater volume than this.

DISCLOSURE OF DONOR

Changes in society are occurring that demand greater freedom of information. One of these may be that in future, a child from a pregnancy which started with DI may wish to know the identity of the donor. If this is made law, the donor must give his consent before giving his first semen sample. Short of this, confidentiality must be kept and the clinic must keep information about donors and recipients separately, but be capable of linking.

ADOPTION

In cases of intractable infertility adoption may be considered although there is a great shortage of babies for adoption in the Western world.

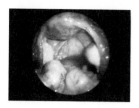

Screening for gynaecological cancer

Cervix, 209
  Current position, 209
  Taking a smear, 210
  Examination of the
    smear, 212
  Grading the smears, 213
  Effectiveness of cervical
    screening, 213
Benefits of cervical
  screening, 215
Ovary, 216

CERVIX

The best known screening service is for squamous cell carcinoma of the cervix which should be a preventable disease because:
- there is usually a phase of premalignancy or dysplasia;
- the cervix is a relatively accessible organ to examine;
- cells can be easily obtained and examined in the premalignant phases.

The biggest problem is access to the population of women liable to develop a carcinoma of the cervix to perform the screening.

Current position

In the UK screening is aimed at all women at risk from within five years of starting sexual activity (usually 15 to 20 years) to the age of 65 years. After this the development of premalignant lesions is extremely rare.

The screening service for cervical cancer is still not operating efficiently but aims to recall women at the correct intervals. It is possible that some carcinomas will grow very rapidly, but for the majority a cervical smear performed every three years will pick up the pathological warning signs. Three yearly smears would detect 91% of the premalignant conditions. Increasing the smear frequency to yearly would only improve the pick-up rate to 93%; so by trebling the work load the improvement would be only 2%.

Smear tests are offered at most places where women attend for obstetric or gynaecological procedures. Thus they may be done at:
- GP surgeries;
- antenatal clinics;
- family planning clinics;

- Genito-Urinary Medicine clinics;
- gynaecology out-patient clinics;
- well-woman clinics.

Since the average age group of those with premalignant conditions is older than the reproductive age group, the most appropriate place for smear tests is the GP surgery, provided that there is a well organized system for recall. This probably means a computer generated record system using an age-sex register with some method of ensuring that those who do not accept their invitation are followed up. There must also be some system of ensuring that the results are returned to the woman reasonably promptly.

This requires an enthusiastic general practitioner service which is appropriately funded. In the UK, recent changes in the National Health Service offer incentives to general practitioners to achieve targets of ensuring a high percentage of those in the higher risk age groups receive their smears at correct intervals.

Taking a smear

The smear can be taken by anyone competent to perform a vaginal examination; thus it can be done by a gynaecologist, a general practitioner, a local authority clinic doctor, a trained midwife or a nurse.

After discussion, the woman is positioned on the couch and a warmed speculum is passed to expose the cervix. There is much debate as to whether a digital vaginal assessment should be made before the speculum is passed, in order to ensure that the correct size of speculum is used. It is probable that for most women who are having intercourse (i.e., most of the population who attend for cervical smears) a medium sized speculum will be suitable. If a digital examination is performed before passing the speculum, it reassures the woman, for a finger is smaller and less unyielding than a metal speculum. However, care should be taken not to rub the finger on the cervix for this could remove surface cells which should appear on the smear.

When the cervix has been exposed, a spatula is used to scrape the whole squamo-columnar junction. If the external os is regular, the pointed end of a spatula can be passed into the canal and rotated by 360° (Fig. 17.1). If the cervical os is irregular or gaping, the blunt end of the spatula should be used (Fig. 17.2). New spatulae are being developed each year and the most commonly used is the Aylesbury spatula with its elongated beak to go up the cervical canal.

The material removed on the tip of the spatula should be rapidly smeared onto a clean glass slide and fixed immediately. It is important that the fixing agent is used straight away to prevent the cells drying in

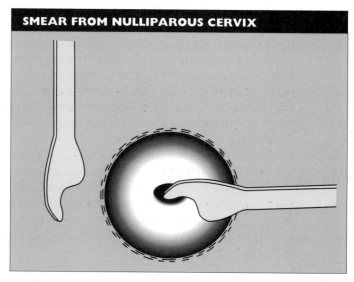

Fig. 17.1 Smear taken from a nulliparous cervix with the shaped end of an Ayre's spatula.

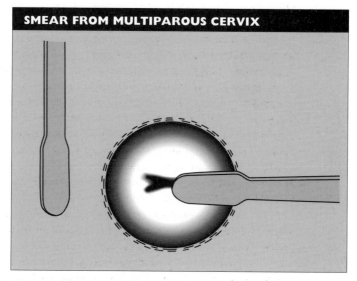

Fig. 17.2 Smear taken from a multiparous cervix with the rounded end of an Ayre's spatula.

air. The name of the patient and number should have been written on the slide before smearing so it can go straight into the fixative medium or be sprayed with the fixative aerosol. The alcohol/ether mixture dries rapidly fixing the cell and nuclei. The slide can then be kept in a container to go to the laboratory either through the post or by messenger.

The cytopathologist will need certain basic information about the woman in order that the findings can be interpreted more carefully.

- The age of the woman.
- Woman's occupation.
- Partner's occupation.
- Menstrual cycle and date of last menstrual period.
- Is she pregnant?
- Any current hormone therapy (including oral contraception)?
- Presence of intrauterine device.
- State of the cervix.

Examination of the smear

It is not the best time to take a smear during menstruation for red cells obscure the epithelial cells in microscopic examination of the smear. However, if the woman has irregular bleeding from a cervical lesion it is impossible to avoid this. A note should be made to the pathologist if this occurs.

At the laboratory the smear is stained and examined by cytotechnicians. If any abnormality is detected, the smear will be passed to a cytopathologist.

False negative results
Where a woman actually has premalignant changes in her cells but these are not reported. Incidence is unknown but from data on women who do develop carcinoma of the cervix, it is probably between 10 and 30%. Causes include:

- error in taking the smear:
    (a) non-representative sample of cells;
    (b) not from squamo-columnar junction;
- a misinterpretation in the laboratory itself;
- incorrect typing of the report from the laboratory.

False positive results
Where the smear is reported as having a greater degree of malignant change than exists. This is caused by:

- misinterpretion by the cytologist;
- infection;

- pregnancy;
- incorrect typing of results on the report.

Grading the smears

The classical grading of cervical smears is the Papanicolaou classification:
Stage 1—normal cells only.
Stage 2—inflammatory cells with normal cells.
Stage 3—inflammatory plus a few mildly suspicious cells.
Stage 4—cells suspicious of malignancy.
Stage 5—malignant cells.

This has mostly been superseded by the cervical intraepithelial neoplasia classification (CIN) which started as a histological classification grading the type of cells seen at a histological biopsy. It has now developed into a histological classification grading the depth of changes in the epithelium seen at biopsy. Some cytopathologists now interpret cervical smears on a CIN classification finding the cells coming from different depths of the epithelium:
CIN I—normal cells seen.
CIN II—some suspicious cells only. Probably infective.
CIN III—frankly malignant cells seen.

In practice, a description of the cell changes seen is more valuable than any numbers allocated by various grading systems.

Effectiveness of cervical screening

If cervical screening were totally effective, carcinoma of the cervix would be eliminated. Approximately 2000 women still die annually from this condition in the UK so the cervical screening programme has obviously not been so effective. Countries with a more extensive cervical screening programme than the UK's report a diminution in deaths from carcinoma of the cervix (Fig. 17.3).

No screening programme can have perfect success in controlling disease because:
- screening may not reach all the population at risk;
- there will be false negatives;
- the infrequency of screening may miss a rapidly progressive case;
- treatment as a result of screening may be incorrectly given;
- the treatment that follows screening may not be effective;
- recurrences may occur after even apparently successful courses of treatment.

Screening in the UK is not uniform. It has been opportunistic, mostly being performed at places where women attend. The only way to make

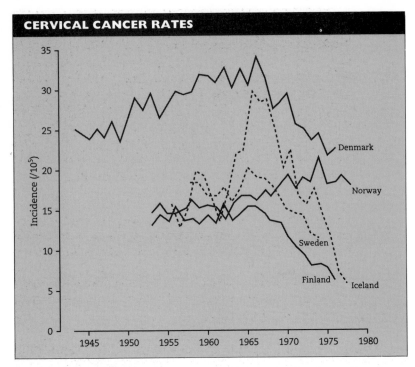

CERVICAL CANCER RATES

Fig. 17.3 Incidence of cervical cancer in the Nordic countries. Norway was the only country with no cervical cancer screening programme.

CERVICAL SCREENING—BENEFITS AND DRAWBACKS

Advantages

1 Reassurance for most who have no premalignant changes

2 Reassurance to a few that any premalignant changes found are at a very early stage

3 Avoidance of radical treatments if the condition is picked up early

4 Produce an increased life expectancy

Disadvantages

1 Fear of finding cancer. This may sound illogical but it is true for most human beings

2 The anxiety generated while waiting for the results

3 The fear that comes from false positive results

Box 17.1 The benefits and drawbacks to the individual woman of cervical screening.

CERVICAL SCREENING FREQUENCIES— COSTS AND BENEFITS

Interval	Positive smears (%)	Approx no. smears taken in life	Approx annual costs of screening (£ million)
5 yearly	84	10	50
Going to 3 yearly	91	17	85
Going to 1 yearly	93	51	250

Table 17.1 The cost/benefits of different frequencies of cervical smears.

it work properly will be to have a full GP based programme with recall systems and a check of those not attending. At present, the majority of women in the UK who die of clinical carcinoma had never had a cervical smear at all.

Rapidly progressive cases are rare, but women who have had a carcinoma of the cervix can have had a normal smear performed within a year or so, but this is unusual.

Benefits of cervical screening

A screening programme should aim to benefit the individual first (Box 17.1) and then society.

Society however can reap benefits or disadvantages from extending the cervical screening programme. If priority is given to cervical screening, monies have to be diverted from other resources and other services curtailed.

The cost/benefits of different aspects of cervical cancer screening can be assessed; an example is the frequency with which smears are taken (Table 17.1). The financial benefits to society of a successful cervical screening programme would be the avoidance of expenditure in treating advanced cancer and the extra years of productivity of people who have survived.

CONCLUSION

In the UK, the cervical screening programme has not in the past been as effective as it might. In order to achieve a three yearly smear for the 20 million women at risk, a more organized system of screening is now provided, but will take a decade to come into full effect.

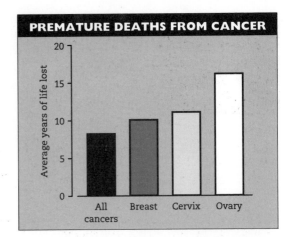

Fig. 17.4 Average premature deaths from different cancers.

OVARY

Cancer of the ovary is a significant cause of premature death in women, before the expected age of 75 (Fig. 17.4). It is often diagnosed late because of its lack of symptoms and it commonly metastasizes quickly and widely (Chapter 8). Hence, a screening test would be helpful. At present, two methods are possible.

- Serum marker CA125:

    (a) 25% of those with ovarian carcinoma are positive five years before clinical diagnosis;

    (b) 50% of those with ovarian carcinoma are positive one and a half years before clinical diagnosis.

- Ultrasound—high sensitivity for ovarian tumours, but:

    (a) invasive;

    (b) depends on experience and equipment which is not universally available;

    (c) needs expert ultrasonographers who are not available in all Health Authorities and Trusts.

Hence, use CA125 as first screen and ultrasound as backup screen. Even a modest increase in earlier diagnosis could reduce death rates considerably.

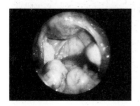

Contraception

Trends, 217
Counselling, 218
  Methods used by the female, 219
  Methods used by the male, 220
  Methods used by both partners, 220

Hormones: oral contraceptives, 220
Combined pill, 220
Emergency pill (post coital contraception), 224
Progestogen-only pill, 224
Injectable contraceptives, 225

Intrauterine devices, 225
Barrier contraception, 229
Chemical contraceptives, 230
Douching, 231
Methods used by the male, 231
Methods used by both partners, 232

Contraception is the use of techniques to prevent pregnancy while allowing intercourse to continue. The ideal contraceptive should be safe, harmless and not interfere with the sexual enjoyment of either party.

Distinguish between family planning and population control.

• *Family planning*, a personal matter demanding a low failure rate and

• *Population control* where the need for cheapness and ease of use may make a less exacting standard of efficacy acceptable.

The failure rate of any method of contraception is judged by the Pearl Index (PI); the number of women having regular intercourse who become pregnant within a year out of 100 couples using the method.

$$PI = \frac{\text{number of pregnancies}}{\text{number of couples using the method}} \times 100$$

Sterilization (Chapter 19) and termination of pregnancy (Chapter 20) are both methods of family limitation, but they are not reversible and so strictly are not contraception.

TRENDS

Contraception has been available in the UK for several centuries, mostly in the form of barrier methods in the earlier days. In the 1960s the hormonal method and intrauterine devices (IUDs) became popular. In the 1970s, free family planning was available from the National Health Service. This led to an increase in availability and uptake of all methods in

WHO DATA ON CONTRACEPTIVES BY PERCENTAGE

	Oral contraceptives	Intruterine device	Sheath	Other methods	Sterilization Male	Sterilization Female
Developed regions	13	6	13	27	4	7
Developing regions	6	10	3	6	5	15
World	8	9	5	11	5	13

Table 18.1 Data on contraceptives by percentages. World Health Organization, 1989.

all groups of age, sex or marital status. In the 1970s doubts were raised about the risks of hormonal contraception which by the 1980s had been resolved somewhat only to be followed by the fears of HIV which led to the wider use of the condom for safer sex. At the same time, the long-lasting IUDs came on the market and offered less intrusion upon sexual life. In the mid 1990s long-lasting injectables are also becoming more widely used. Table 18.1 shows the World Health Organization (WHO) data in 1989 of various usages in types of regions.

Sterilization also has increased in popularity since the late 1970s so that about a quarter of couples choose this as their method.

COUNSELLING

Family planning and birth control need discussion of more than just the mechanics of methods. They are part of reproductive life linked with emotional and sexual life. There is sometimes embarrassment surrounding family planning and so this matter is not discussed openly. For example, contraceptive advertising is not accepted on the London Underground, but is at the airport. It is for professionals to try and help break these barriers by discussing the matter in a clear and simple fashion.

The use of contraception is influenced by many factors other than just the regulation of reproduction. These include:

- cultural background;
- religion;
- partnership status;
- personal health;
- personal habits.

The influence of peer comments is probably even greater than that of professionals. If a woman has met someone who had a bad time on the pill, this will be remembered more than advice given by the family

CHECK LIST OF CONTRACEPTIVE COUNSELLING

When discussing any methods of contraception consider:
- suitability
- side-effects
- risks
- benefits
- how it works
- after sales service
- professionals

Box 18.1 Check list of contraceptive counselling.

planner. When counselling, the professionals should listen quite as much as they should advise. There are not enough data available on the use of methods to be absolute. The failure rate is not the only thing that influences people. When counselling, the items in Box 18.1 should all be included. The provision of contraception is one of the most intimate areas of an individual's life and requires high skills in communication and information giving.

Methods used by the female

HORMONAL
- The pill—combined oral contraceptive (oestrogen and progestogen).
- The emergency pill—high dose oestrogen with progestogen.
- The mini-pill—progestogen-only pills.
- Injectable hormones—progestogens.
- Implantable hormones—progestogens.

INTRAUTERINE DEVICES (IUDS)

BARRIERS TO OCCLUDE THE CERVIX
- Diaphragm or Dutch cap.
- Cervical cap.
- Vault pessary.
- Vaginal sheath.

CHEMICAL SPERMICIDES
- Soluble pessaries.
- Creams, foams and jellies.

- Medicated sponges.
- Douching.

Methods used by the male

- The sheath, condom or French letter.
- Withdrawal or coitus reservatus.
- Male pill.

Methods used by both partners

- Intercourse without penetration.
- Periodic intercourse using the safe period.
- Abstinence.

HORMONES: ORAL CONTRACEPTIVES

Combined pill

The pill is used by about a third of women in the UK who use contraception. There is a wide range of oral contraceptives (Table 18.2). Most are a mixture of an oestrogen taken for 21 days out of the 28 and a progestogen used for the last 7 to 10 days of the cycle. The pill probably:
- inhibits ovulation by interfering with gonadotrophin releasing hormones;
- modifies the endometrium preventing implantation;
- makes the cervical secretion more viscid and less permeable to spermatozoa.

ADVANTAGES

- The pill is the most effective method of birth control provided the instructions are followed and it is taken regularly.
- The method is not related to the act of intercourse.
- Women who suffer from dysmenorrhoea or heavy periods often find their periods less painful and the flow diminished.
- Menstruation occurs at regular intervals of four weeks.
- Haemoglobin levels are maintained so that anaemia is less common.

METABOLIC EFFECTS

In different women there maybe as much as a 10-fold variation in tissue levels of the hormones and therefore of their effects because of:
- difference in absorption;

EXAMPLES OF ORAL CONTRACEPTIVES

Pill type	Preparation	Oestrogen (µg)	Progestogen (mg)	
Combined				
Ethinyloestradiol/	Lestrin 20	20	1	
norethisterone	Loestrin 30	30	1.5	
	Brevinor	35	0.5	
	Norimin	35	1	
Ethinyloestradiol/	Microgynon 30	30	0.15	
levonorgestrel	Eugynon 30	30	0.25	
	Ovran	50	2.25	
Ethinyloestradiol/	Marvelon	30	0.15	
desogestrel				
Ethinyloestradiol/	Femodene	30	0.075	
gestodene				
Ethinyloestradiol/	Cilest	35	0.25	
norgestimate				
Ethinyloestradiol/	Norinyl-1	50	1	
norethisterone	Ortho-Novin 1/50	50	1	
Biphasic	BiNovum	35	0.5	(7 tabs)
		35	1	(14 tabs)
Triphasic	TriNovum	35	0.5	(7 tabs)
		35	0.75	(7 tabs)
		35	1	(7 tabs)
Ethinyloestradiol/	Trinordiol	30	0.05	(6 tabs)
levonorgestrel		40	0.075	(5 tabs)
		30	0.125	(10 tabs)
Ethinyloestradiol/	Tri-Minulet	30	0.05	(6 tabs)
gestodene		40	0.07	(5 tabs)
		30	0.1	(10 tabs)
Progestogen ONLY				
Norethisterone	Noriday	–	0.35	norethisterone
	Femulen	–	0.5	ethynodiol diacetate
Levonorgestrel	Microval	–	0.03	
	Neogest	–	0.075	norgestrel

Table 18.2 Some examples of oral contraceptives in current use in the UK.

- difference in liver metabolism of steroids;
- difference in fat layers of body as fat adsorbs steroids avidly.
    Glucose tolerance may be impaired.
    There may be an increase in:
- low density lipo-proteins;
- cholesterol;
- serum iron;
- serum copper;
- circulating blood coagulation factors VII, IX;
- fibrinogen.

SIDE-EFFECTS

- There may be fluid retention and weight gain.
- Break-through bleeding may occur in the first cycle and later if the amount of oestrogen is too low.
- Thrombo-embolism may occur, but mainly with high oestrogen dosage.
- Skin pigmentation rather like the chloasma of pregnancy may develop.
- Acne may recur; migraine may be aggravated.
- Depression occurs in a few.
- There is a little evidence that the pill is carcinogenic to the cervix or the breast. Much of this relates to the higher dose oestrogens and progestogens used in oral contraceptives (OC) 10 years ago.
- There is lower incidence of cancer of the ovary (by 40%) and endo-metrium (by 50%).

CONTRA-INDICATIONS

- The most serious hazards are:
    (a) thrombo-embolism;
    (b) coronary thrombosis;
    (c) cerebrovascular accident.
- The pill should be avoided in women:
    (a) with a history or family history of thrombo-phlebitis, varicose veins, or severe heart disease;
    (b) over 40 if they are obese and smoke heavily;
    (c) with liver damage including recent infective hepatitis or glandular fever;
    (d) with a history of breast cancer;
    (e) with excess weight, more than 50% of ideal;
    (f) with moderate hypertension;
    (g) with true sickle cell disease-genotype SS or SC (but not sickle trait, Genotype AS).
    Women taking the pill who undergo surgery face an increased risk

of thrombosis and embolism during the post-operative period. The pill should ideally be stopped six weeks before elective surgery and immediately in the case of illness or accidents leading to long immobilization.

DRUG INTERACTIONS

Certain drugs may interfere with the absorption, metabolism or efficacy of oral contraceptives.

- Phenytoin.
- Barbiturates.
- Anti-tuberculous drugs (e.g., rifampicin).
- Antibiotics (e.g., griseofulvin and tetracycline).

The dose of hypoglycaemic agents may need increasing while the effect of corticosteroids may be enhanced. Epileptic women may need double the normal oral contraceptive dose to inhibit breakthrough bleeding and achieve maximum safety if they are on sodium valproate or clonazepam.

PRESCRIBING THE PILL

A careful *history* should be taken with reference to conditions such as heavy smoking which may increase the risk of the pill.

Examination should include a record of blood pressure and body weight. The breasts, heart and abdomen should be examined and a note made of varicose veins. A pelvic examination should be made to exclude a condition such as uterine fibroids which might contra-indicate the pill.

The choice of oral contraception often depends on the individual doctor's preference; the list of available pills is extensive. In general:

- 20 µg pills are best kept for the very slim;
- 50 µg pills are little used now.

Watch for interacting drugs that are also being taken. The choice lies between a 30 or 35 µg pill to be taken either continuously or as one of the biphasic or triphasic pills.

The first pill of the bi- and triphasic course is taken on the first day of menstruation. Successors are either taken for 21 days with seven pill free days during which a withdrawal bleed occurs or continuously depending on the brand. Good instructions come with each packet and should be read.

There may be some side-effects such as early morning nausea, breast tenderness and slight bleeding during the first cycle. The *tricyclic regime* suits some women; here a 35 µg pill, with a varying degree of progestogen is given for 21 days, then 7 pill free days when bleeding should occur. This may help sufferers from migraine or epilepsy and also suits some women who have to travel a great deal.

The combined pill should not be given during lactation, the progestogen-only pill being preferred then. The pill may be started on the second day after an abortion or termination of pregnancy.

The method should be carefully explained and discussed. The woman is advised to report adverse effects immediately. Regular examination with tests for blood pressure, glycosuria and excessive weight gain is essential.

FORGOTTEN PILLS

If a pill is missed, advise the woman to take the missed one as soon as it is realized. If it is within 12 hours of the usual time, contraception is probably secure. If longer than this, the pill may not work. Alternate contraception (i.e., condom) or abstinence is advised for seven days. If the missed OC is the last of the pack, go straight into the next cycle's pack—there will probably be no period but there will be better contraception.

Emergency pill (post coital contraception)

Oestrogen taken in large doses after unprotected coitus and before implantation may prevent pregnancy. Combined preparations containing 50 µg of ethinyloestradiol and 250 µg of levonorgestrel (Ovran or Norinyl-1) may be used in double dose. Two tablets are given immediately and repeated after twelve hours. The main side-effects are nausea and vomiting.

Treatment should be given within 72 hours of a single incident of unprotected intercourse and within three days of predicted ovulation. The old name of morning-after pill is a misnomer. The next period can be early or be late; the woman should have a pregnancy test if she does not menstruate.

Progestogen-only pill

Progestogens are used for oral contraception; they probably act not by inhibiting ovulation but by their effect on the cervical mucus and the endometrium.

The progestogen-only pill is taken continuously at the same time of day from the first day of menstruation. If the pill is delayed more than three hours, additional precautions or abstinence are needed until the pill has been taken continuously for 14 days.

There is a failure rate of 1 to 4 per 100 women/years. There may be irregular bleeding or amenorrhoea and there is a slightly increased risk of thrombosis. They are useful in older women.

Injectable contraceptives

Those most commonly used consist of a progestogen given by intramuscular injection or as subcutaneous implants. They are not the first choice for contraception but are widely used in developing countries and in the UK for women when other methods are unacceptable or contraindicated.

Depo-medroxy-progesterone acetate (Depo-Provera) is given in a dose of 150 mg repeated every 12 weeks or 90 days. Norethisterone enanthate (Noristerat) is given in doses of 200 mg every eight weeks.

Side-effects include weight gain, irregular bleeding and amenorrhoea. They should not be given until six weeks after childbirth.

Silastic capsules injected subcutaneously under local anaesthesia are now available in the UK. Leio-norgestrel implants (Norplant) offer up to five years of protection and can be removed readily when the return of fertility is required. Alternatively, at five years they can be replaced.

INTRAUTERINE DEVICES

Intrauterine devices have existed for centuries, the best known being the Grafenberg ring made of silver or German gold inserted into the uterus.

In recent years devices were made of plastic, one of the better known being the Lippes loop which is rarely seen in the Western world now (Fig. 18.1). These have been superseded in UK practice by devices incorporating copper; some also have a silver core and have extra copper on the horizontal arms. Medico-legal problems in the USA have led to the withdrawal of a number of intrauterine devices. In the UK the following devices are still available, some of which are shown in Fig. 18.2.

Copper devices
- Multiload.
- Cu 250.
- Cu 250 short.
- Cu 375.

Copper devices with silver core
- Novagard.
- Nova-T.
- Ortho-Gyne T (380 Slimline).

Progestogen devices
- Minerva.

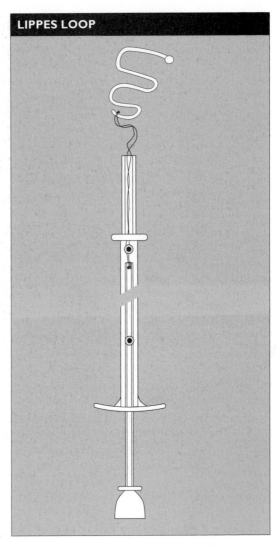

Fig. 18.1 Lippes loop
intrauterine contraception.

ADVANTAGES

An IUD gives permanent protection and requires no attention at the time of intercourse. Provided that there are no complications a device can remain in the uterus for up to five years; in the last decade of reproductive life, this may be extended as potential fertility is less.

DISADVANTAGES

A skilled doctor or nurse is required to insert an IUD. When first inserted there may be pain and bleeding. The menstrual flow may be

INTRAUTERINE DEVICES

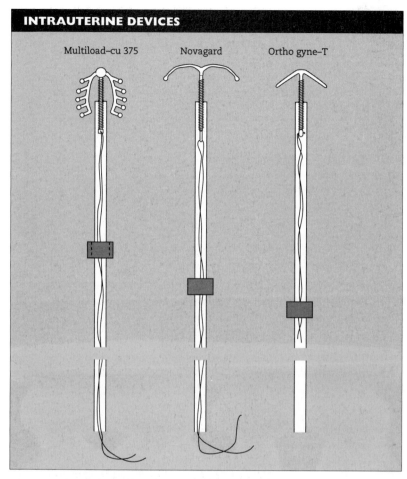

Multiload–cu 375   Novagard   Ortho gyne–T

Fig. 18.2 Some types of intrauterine devices in common use

increased and the periods prolonged for a few months. There is risk of flairing up tubal infection.

COMPLICATIONS

- The device may pass unnoticed, especially during menstruation.
- Pelvic infection may occur.
- Increased risk of rejection in nulliparous women.
- Perforation of the uterus may occur with the coil moving into the peritoneal cavity. This is usually at the time of insertion particularly with an acutely anteflexed or retroflexed uterus. If it occurs with a copper device it must be removed very soon, either by laparoscopy or by laparotomy.

- There is no evidence that intrauterine devices are carcinogenic.
- The thread may disappear. The continued presence of the device can be checked by ultrasound. Removal is usually easy in the out-patients department.
- While the rate of intrauterine pregnancy is reduced, that of ectopics is not. Hence, there is a relative increase in ectopic pregnancy after IUD insertion.

CONTRA-INDICATIONS

An IUD should not be inserted in the presence of:
- pelvic infection;
- uterine fibroids;
- genital malignancy;
- abnormal bleeding;
- menorrhagia.

METHOD OF INSERTION

The device is supplied in a sterile pack with full instructions for insertion. This should be done with aseptic and antiseptic precautions (Fig. 18.3).
- The best time is at the end of menstruation.

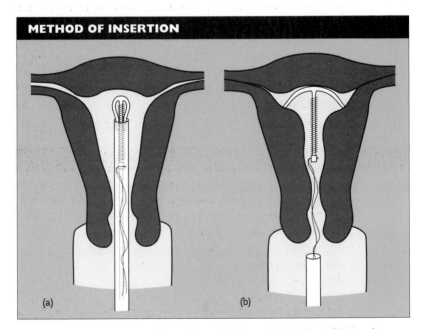

METHOD OF INSERTION

(a)   (b)

Fig. 18.3 (a) The T-shaped IUD is straightened inside a plastic tube and inserted through the cervix. (b) When pushed from the hollow tube it resumes its old shape.

- The cervix is exposed and may be steadied with a single-toothed forceps.
- A sound measures uterine length.
- The device is loaded into the introducer and inserted.
- The introducer is withdrawn and the nylon threads cut leaving 1.5 to 2.0 cm in the upper vagina.
- The woman should be taught to identify the threads.

A vasovagal attack may occur at the time of insertion, following cervical stimulation. This usually responds on stopping the insertion and lowering the woman's head. Formal resuscitation is very rarely needed, but facilities should be available at the family planning clinic for the rare occasion.

POST COITAL CONTRACEPTION

An intrauterine device may be used for post coital contraception to prevent implantation if inserted within five days of unprotected intercourse. The woman must be seen again to ensure menstruation has occurred. This is an emergency measure, but if normal menstruation occurs the device may be left for permanent contraception.

PREGNANCY

The pregnancy rate with copper devices is reported as 1.4 per 100 women/years. Should pregnancy occur the possibility of ectopic pregnancy must be excluded.

- If the tail of the device is visible the device should be removed by pulling gently on the thread.
- If the tail of the device is not found the position of the device must be checked by ultrasound.
- The device may be left in the uterus throughout pregnancy.

BARRIER CONTRACEPTION

The most effective is the *vaginal diaphragm* or Dutch cap which consists of a watch spring or coiled spring edge with a dome of latex (Fig. 18.4). They are made in various sizes and for maximum safety must be used with a spermicide jelly or cream.

- The correct size must be selected before examination (Fig. 18.5).
- The woman taught how to insert and remove it.
- Always use it with a spermicide.
- Leave it in for eight hours after intercourse.
- A check of the fit and if need be refitting after six months, and after childbirth.

If there is prolapse or a retroverted uterus, an alternative is the

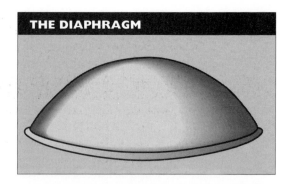

Fig. 18.4 The contraceptive diaphragm.

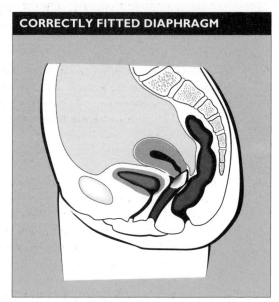

Fig. 18.5 The diaphragm fits snugly to the walls of the vagina occluding the cervix from the rest of the vagina.

cervical cap made of rubber or plastic. This is harder to get in place and easier to displace at intercourse.

The *vaginal sheath* is a plastic bag which lines the vagina. It retains its place by a spring ring in the fornices. The woman can insert it at leisure. It has mixed popularity among women and their partners.

CHEMICAL CONTRACEPTIVES

These are mainly spermicides. They may be bought over the counter and do not need professional advice. Creams, gels, soluble pessaries and foaming preparations exist. The failure rate is relatively high if used alone.

A disposable plastic sponge impregnated with spermicide (nonoxinol-9) can be placed high in the vagina. It is less effective than the diaphragm with a PI of about 9 per 100 women/years.

DOUCHING

Douching immediately after intercourse with warm water or a weak solution of vinegar (one teaspoon to a pint) is a time honoured but ineffective method. It does not affect those sperms which have already passed up the cervical canal.

METHODS USED BY THE MALE

THE SHEATH

The sheath, condom or French letter is one of the commonest methods of contraception. It requires no medical intervention and can be bought in many non-medical places. For maximum safety the woman should insert a chemical contraceptive in case the sheath bursts or slips off. Another advantage is that is reduces the spread of sexually transmitted infections, including HIV.

COITUS INTERRUPTUS

This is the oldest and a widely practised method: the male withdraws before ejaculation. It is not always reliable for human beings are frail. It may prevent complete satisfaction to both partners. In *coitus reservatus* the man enters the vagina but does not ejaculate. This is even more unreliable for who wants to stop?

METHODS USED BY BOTH PARTNERS

THE SAFE PERIOD OR NATURAL FAMILY PLANNING

In theory ovulation occurs only once in each menstrual cycle, so there are days when a woman can expect to be infertile. These can be calculated in various ways.

• The calendar method based on working out the fertile period from previous cycles (Table 18.3).

• The basal temperature method depends on the rise of basal temperature which follows ovulation. Intercourse is stopped for three days before and after ovulation.

• Teaching the woman to note the changes in cervical mucus which occurs at ovulation and marks the peak of fertility. Instead of sticky glue-

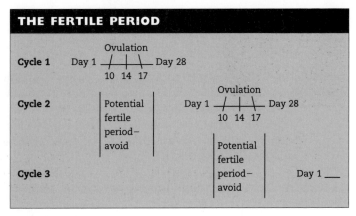

Table 18.3 The fertile time to avoid when using the calendar method of contraception.

like mucus, it becomes thin and runny. Motivation is important as is adequate instruction.

The disadvantage of the safe period is that it is not really safe if menstruation is irregular, after childbirth or abortion or in women approaching the menopause.

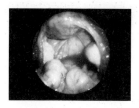

Sterilization

Counselling for
    sterilization, 233
Female sterilization, 233

Laparotomy sterilization,
    234
Laparoscopic
    sterilization, 235

Other methods, 238
Causes of failure, 238
Male sterilization, 239
Procedure, 240

Sterilization is an operation aimed at the permanent occlusion of tubes carrying the gametes.

COUNSELLING FOR STERILIZATION

Sterilization is an important step in the life of any man or woman. With present methods it should be considered as irrevocable for while reversal is possible for both males and females, success cannot be guaranteed even in the most expert hands.

Counselling is important and consent must be given in writing. The consent of the spouse is no longer necessary legally but it is desirable that the couple should be seen together and the full implications of the procedure explained. It has often been found that a request for sterilization may be a cry for help where a marriage is not going well, where there has been a bereavement or a failure of contraception. When obtaining consent, the risks of failure must be made clear and a record of this discussion made in the case notes. These risks vary with the different methods; with female sterilization, as part of the failure, there is the small added risk of ectopic pregnancy—this too should be discussed.

A girl under 16 cannot consent to sterilization, nor can her parents insist on it. The same applies to individuals who are mentally retarded to a degree that they cannot understand the meaning and consequences of the operation. At present such operations can only be performed with the consent of a High Court judge.

FEMALE STERILIZATION

The most practical place to block the female genital tract is at the fallopian tubes. These are deep inside the peritoneal cavity, so their approach is a bigger procedure than operating on the male. The use of the laparoscope has reduced much of the need for large incisions in the majority of cases but it is still an operation inside the peritoneal cavity requiring a general anaesthetic and the availability of full surgical skills.

Laparotomy sterilization

This is done at a full laparotomy and involves a general anaesthesia and relaxation. The woman should plan to stay in hospital for two to five days depending on how fit she is.

The simplest operation was described by Pomeroy and is shown in Fig. 19.1. It is not often performed now. A more common technique is the Irving method, where each tube is divided and separated. The medial end is implanted in a tunnel in the wall of the uterus (Fig. 19.2).

The operation of formal surgical division is commonly performed these days whilst doing a Caesarean section when the abdomen is open. The failure rate is about 0.2 per hundred women/years.

A lesser abdominal operation (Mini-Lap) can be performed by an experienced surgeon. A 5 cm transverse suprapubic incision is extended to the rectus sheath and the surgeon then separates the rectus muscles. This allows a bivalve speculum to be introduced through the incision into the peritoneal cavity. Through this, each fallopian tube in turn can be sought, drawn up and operated upon. It is divided and the two ends

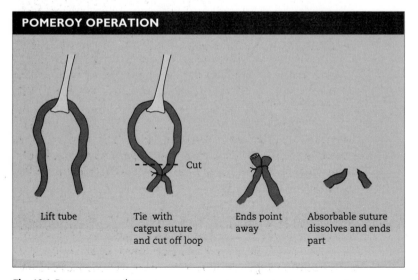

POMEROY OPERATION

Lift tube

Tie with catgut suture and cut off loop

Cut

Ends point away

Absorbable suture dissolves and ends part

Fig. 19.1 Pomeroy operation.

IRVING OPERATION

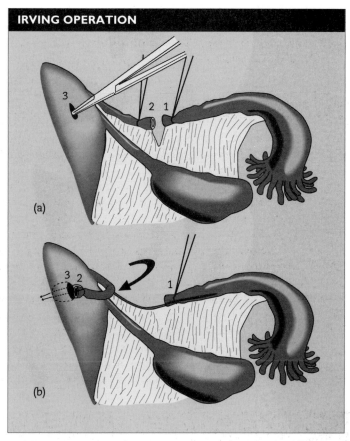

Fig. 19.2 Irving method. The diagrams (a) and (b) show the principles of the operation. The tube is divided (1) and its medial end (2) is implanted in a tunnel (3) in the wall of the uterus. This method ought to be foolproof. In the very few occasions it has failed it must be suspected that the surgeon's technique was faulty.

overlapped so that the ends are separated (Fig. 19.3). This operation is often done in developing countries where laparoscopy is not readily available. The failure rate for this operation is about 1 to 2 per 1000 operations.

Laparoscopic sterilization

This operation is performed through a small incision but is potentially just as hazardous as a larger operation. It should only be performed by those who are skilled in general gynaecological surgery because the abdomen

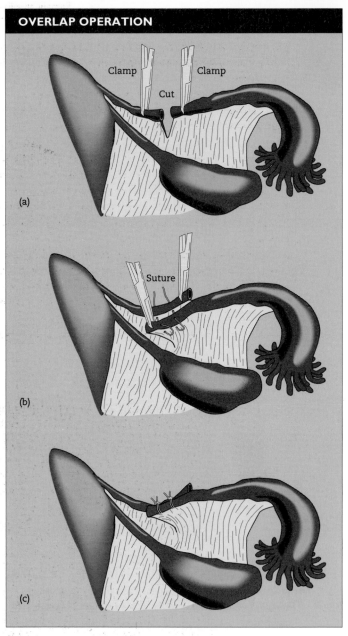

Fig. 19.3 Female sterilization. (a) At laparotomy, each tube is doubly clamped and divided between the clamps. (b) The two broad ends are overlapped and two sutures run through the overlapping leaves of the broad ligament underneath the tubes. (c) The sutures are tied and the clamps removed. Thus each tube has crushed areas ligated, has been divided and the two ends face in different ways separated by 3 cm of peritonial cavity.

may have to be opened at any time to deal with complications. These are however uncommon and often the laparoscopic sterilization can be done as a day case.

The tube is then blocked by one of three methods.

1 A *mechanical clip* (Hulka–Clemens, Filshie) may be applied to each tube. This may be a spring-loaded clip or a plastic one with a grip (Fig. 19.4).

2 A *silastic ring* (Falope ring) may be applied to the medial narrow part of each tube through the laparoscope (Fig. 19.5). A knuckle of tube is drawn up and over it is slipped a silastic ring which constricts the neck of the knuckle. This causes necrosis of the tube at the bound point, which then fibroses blocking the lumen and then pulls apart leaving the tube with a gap.

3 *Unipolar or bipolar diathermy* can be used to cauterize the fallopian tube in two places about 1 cm apart in the isthmal area. There is a slight risk of the heat damaging a nearby organ, such as the bowel. Furthermore, it is very difficult to reverse this operation. For these reasons, it is less commonly used in the Western world.

Failure rates of laparoscopic sterilizations are about 1 to 2 per 1000 operations.

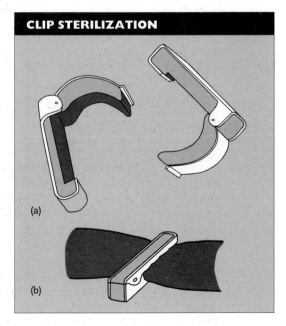

CLIP STERILIZATION

(a)

(b)

Fig. 19.4 (a) A clip and (b) its method of application.

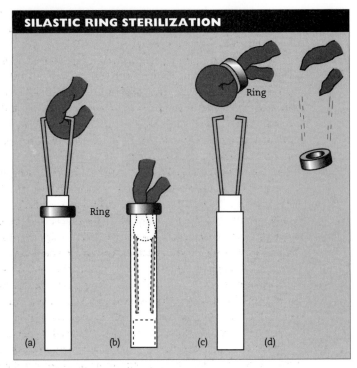

Fig. 19.5 A silastic ring and its method of application. (a) The springy forceps grasp the tube. (b) Retracting the forceps draws the tube through the plastic ring. (c) Passing the forceps back releases the tube and the tube is constricted at its neck by the ring. (d) The loop becomes apexic, dies and the ends separate when the ring drops off.

Other methods

Transuterine methods of sterilization without anaesthesia are being attempted through the hysteroscope and passing catheters under ultrasound control through the uterine cavity into the fallopian tubes. A variety of rapidly setting plastic resins have been injected; alternately, electrical cautery or cryosurgery by narrow cooling probes have been used by the same route. None of these methods has yet been shown to produce reliable results.

Causes of failure

Despite these operations, a woman may still get pregnant in 1 to 3 per 1000 cases in the UK.

• The woman may already have a fertilized oocyte in the proximal tube or even the uterus at the time of the operation. Hence most endeavour to operate in the first two weeks of cycle; as a precaution, many perform a uterine curettage at the same time.

• The occluding clip or ring may be correctly placed but springs off or breaks after the operator has left the abdomen. Unless a good knuckle of tube is brought through the elastic ring, it may not be pinching it securely. The clip may re-open under pressure of the tissues although this is less common with the beaked Filshie clip. Very rarely sterilization clips have broken. Thus they have no occlusive effect on the fallopian tube and have been removed subsequently from the abdomen in pieces.

• Although the tube is blocked by the clip and the short length of fibrosis it causes, the two ends of the tube may not separate. A small fistula can form between the contiguous ends bypassing the occluding device or burrowing through the short length of fibrous tissue. This would allow sperm to pass up readily although fertilized eggs might pass down less commonly; in consequence an ectopic pregnancy may result.

• The occluding device may be put on the wrong structure. Laparoscopic sterilization should be done only when the surgeon has good vision. Occasionally, however, with less than perfect sight, a clip is put on the round ligament just in front of the fallopian tube.

A hysterosalpingogram is occasionally performed 16 weeks after the operation to ensure tubal blockage. It is unwise to do it before this as the pressure of the injected dye may disrupt healing tissues and produce a fistula between the blocked parts of the tube.

MALE STERILIZATION

Blockage is performed by division of each vas deferens in the groin, a lesser surgical operation than for the female, but it seems to carry

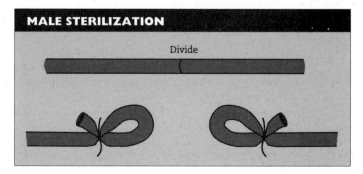

Fig. 19.6 Male sterilization. Divided ends of the vas deferens are turned back and ligated to ensure that the open ends are not just separated but point in opposite directions.

greater psychological overtones. Men have fears of lost libido and of reduced masculinity; these often lurk in the subconscious of the man who will not discuss them. It must be explained that neither usually occurs. Most of the volume of semen is still produced from the prostate gland and it is only the sperm cells that are missing from it. The act of intercourse is exactly the same as before.

Procedure

The operation is usually performed under local anaesthetic in a place where the man can lie down afterwards for an hour. It is often done in the day case theatres of hospitals.

Division and even excision of a piece of tube is not reliable enough for it is very difficult to seal the end of any anatomical tube. When mucosa is close to mucosa, a fistula is often made and so reanastomosis follows. In consequence, the tube is divided and then turned back (Fig. 19.6).

The man should be advised to rest in order to avoid a haematoma. Intercourse is probably best postponed for a week or so to avoid any ache at the site of the wound. Previously used contraceptive methods must be continued for at least three months until all the sperm already in the seminal vesicles have been expelled. This process might be accelerated by flushing out the vas and seminal vesicles with 20 ml of sterile saline during the operation before ligation.

The man must continue ejaculating two or three times a week after the operation to expel the last sperms. A seminal analysis should be performed at two months after the operation. If this is negative and backed by a second negative seminal analysis, then unguarded intercourse may occur. There is a failure rate of between 1 and 4 per 1000 operations.

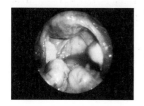

Termination of pregnancy

Position in the UK, 241
Methods, 243
  Early abortion, 244

Mid-trimester abortion,
  245
Later terminations, 246

Menstrual extraction, 246
Medical termination, 247

Pregnancy may be terminated prematurely by interference with the conceptus; this is by intervention with instruments or by drugs. If done incorrectly, there is a high risk of trauma and death of the mother. It is illegal in some societies, but many sovereign States have now passed laws which allow a termination to be performed by doctors under certain constraints.

Religious and cultural factors dictate whether termination is used in a country. Generally, among the Christian religion, termination of pregnancy is unacceptable to the Roman Catholic Church. It is also not accepted by Moslems and some other major world religions. In actuality, it is performed to some degree world-wide irrespective of the official religion or laws of a country.

In some countries, termination of pregnancy is used as a part of the contraceptive programme; in Eastern Europe, up to a third of women use termination as their primary means of contraception. In most of the Western world, this is not so, for it is appreciated that termination of pregnancy has a different order of magnitude of complications than the more conventional methods of contraception.

Four factors have recently rendered it safer in Western society.
• Better training of doctors in the anatomy and physiology of the female genital tract.
• Safe general anaesthesia.
• Asepsis and antisepsis have reduced infection.
• Liberalization of abortion laws encouraging those who want a termination to seek trained medical advice early.

POSITION IN UK

Major changes in the termination of pregnancy were associated with the 1967 Abortion Act (which does not apply in Northern Ireland) and the

EXTRACTS FROM THE ABORTION ACT 1991

A The continuance of the pregnancy would involve risk to the life of the pregnant woman greater than if the pregnancy were terminated

B The termination is necessary to prevent grave permanent injury to the physical or mental health of the pregnant woman

C The pregnancy has NOT exceeded its 24th week and that the continuance of the pregnancy would involve risk, greater than if the pregnancy were terminated, of injury to the physical or mental health of the pregnant woman

D The pregnancy has NOT exceeded its 24th week and that the continuance of the pregnancy would involve risk, greater than if the pregnancy were terminated, of injury to the physical or mental health of any existing child(ren) of the family of the pregnant woman

E There is a substantial risk that if the child were born it would suffer from such physical or mental abnormalities as to be seriously handicapped

Box 20.1 Extracts from the Abortion Act Certificate A (1991).

subsequent 1990 amendment. Before then, terminations had been under an *obiter dictum* or case law which said that a physician may recommend a pregnancy be terminated if he thought that the continuation of pregnancy would harm the mother's physical or mental health. Since the 1967 Abortion Act, the position has been codified into statute law. This was modified in 1990 so that now there are five indications which must be certified in advance by two doctors who should have seen and examined the woman. These are reproduced in Box 20.1, taken from the Abortion Act Certificate A.

In addition, in an emergency, one doctor alone may recommend termination of pregnancy to save the woman's life or health. This indication is very rarely used.

In England and Wales, the various indications are used in the following proportions:

	%
A	0.1
B	2.0
C	88.6
D	8.7
E	0.6
Emergency	<0.01

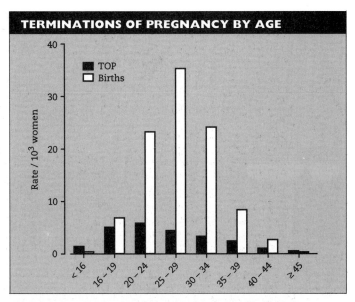

Fig. 20.1 Terminations of pregnancy by age compared with births.

Assessment of the data by age is shown in Fig. 20.1 along with the proportion of births reported in these age groups. There is a shift to the younger women for distribution of terminations.

Most terminations of pregnancy in Britain take place before the 12th week of pregnancy (90%) and few are performed after the 20th week (2.5%) even though the law at present allows this up to the 24th completed week of pregnancy in certain cases. A legal termination of pregnancy must be notified by the operating surgeon to the appropriate Department of Health in England, Scotland or Wales.

METHODS

Any woman presenting with a request for a termination of pregnancy should be assessed carefully. Her GP may know the circumstances of the family well, but the hospital doctor will not. The alternative to abortion is continuation of the pregnancy and its sequelae must be considered:
- adoption;
- placing child with foster parents;
- the mother's parents taking the child.

Usually none of these are acceptable and the woman wishes to go on with the abortion. The GP usually sends her on to a gynaecologist for a second opinion and action, having signed the first half of the consent form.

In the hospital, if in agreement with the GP, the specialist signs the second part. The woman should be checked for fitness for the operation under anaesthesia and some agreement reached about the future method of contraception to avoid a repeat unwanted pregnancy. Many women come as day case admissions especially those seen in the earlier weeks of gestation (before 14 weeks). Termination must be performed in a National Health Hospital or clinic specifically licensed for the purpose.

Early abortion

For pregnancies up to 12 weeks gestation, termination is by a vacuum aspiration of the uterine cavity. A hollow plastic catheter is passed through the cervix which has been gently dilated, sometimes after prostaglandin ripening. A vacuum suction then removes the uterine contents and a gentle curettage ensures the uterus is empty. This technique has a low complication rate and a high success rate.

COMPLICATIONS OF EARLY TERMINATION OF PREGNANCY

Haemorrhage—the uterus in pregnancy is a very vascular organ and separation of the sac and forming placenta causes blood loss. Syntometrine is often needed intravenously to assist the myometrium clamp down on the blood vessels supplying the lining of the uterus.

Perforation—if the uterus is perforated, laparotomy with examination and repair of the uterus may be required.

Infection—termination of pregnancy is an invasive procedure, passing instruments through a potentially septic area (the upper vagina) into a sterile area (the cavity of the uterus). The operator cleans the upper vagina with antiseptic such as chlorhexidine before starting. Antibiotics may be given before the operation if vaginal infection is suspected.

Infection is rare; if it occurs it must be treated promptly with antibiotics or a tubal infection may follow leading to future infertility.

Incomplete termination—this leads to retention of products of conception. Bleeding occurs and re-evacuation of the uterus is necessary.

Psychological complications—many women have a natural grief reaction after early termination of pregnancy; if the abortion was voluntary, that reaction passes in a few weeks or months. Should the woman have been coerced into termination, the reaction can continue for much longer; up to 25% of women in this latter group require psychotherapy.

FUTURE PREGNANCIES

Early termination usually has no effect on future pregnancies. If the cervix is properly dilated to the correct diameter (usually not more than 8mm), there should be no cervical incompetence following early termination of pregnancy which is more commonly found after 10 to 12 mm dilatation.

Mid-trimester abortion

After 14 weeks of gestation, pregnancy termination becomes more difficult.

MORCELLATION AND EXTRACTION

In the hands of an expert and experienced gynaecologist, under anaesthesia the cervix can be dilated to well beyond 10 mm. Crushing instruments are introduced into the uterus to break up the fetus which is then extracted piecemeal. This is an unpleasant and potentially hazardous way to abort, but in expert hands it does mean the whole procedure is over in a few minutes with the mother asleep and unaware of the abortion. She often goes home later the same day.

PROSTAGLANDINS

The uterus can be made to contract by giving prostaglandins ($PGE_{2\alpha}$) per vaginam, intra-amniotically, extra-amniotically or intravenously. The first is the most commonly used method. Under sterile conditions, an amniocentesis is performed drawing 20 ml of amniotic fluid. In its place, 40 mg of $PGE_{2\alpha}$ and 20 ml of super-saturated urea are injected in the amniotic cavity. The former causes the uterus to contract, the latter destroys the placenta and so progesterone levels drop very rapidly, rendering the myometrium more susceptible to the prostaglandins.

A mini-labour follows and delivery usually takes place in 10 to 20 hours. This is painful and so should be well covered with analgesia, maybe an epidural. Evacuation of the placenta is needed in many cases.

HYSTEROTOMY

If prostaglandins are not available, pregnancies after about 14 weeks require a surgical termination and a mini-Caesarean section is performed. There is no lower segment and so the uterine incision has to be vertical. This is rarely done in the UK now.

COMPLICATIONS

Bleeding—this is not common after prostaglandin termination of pregnancy, for the uterus has been contracting through the mini-labour. However, the uterus can be torn by an over-rapid delivery and this may lead to bleeding. The placenta is often retained in terminations between 14 and 22 weeks of pregnancy and usually requires removal under general anaesthesia.

Bleeding is not a major problem after hysterotomy for it is a surgical procedure at which haemostasis is achieved at the time of the operation.

Infection — infection is not common after mid-trimester abortion procedures and should be prevented as it is in any labour or surgical operation by good asepsis and antisepsis.

Psychological problems — such morbidity is greater after mid-trimester abortion. The woman has been pregnant for a longer period and the fetus is more developed. This is an area of great sensitivity which the attendants must be very careful in handling. Some people wish to bury the fetus with a religious service; these natural reactions should be assisted.

Future pregnancies — following mid-trimester abortion, the cervix has been dilated and cervical incompetence can follow. A vertical hysterotomy scar on the uterus might cause a problem, for it is much more liable to rupture in a subsequent pregnancy than a lower segment transverse incision.

Later terminations

Until 1990, termination of pregnancy was only permitted in England, Wales and Scotland before 28 weeks, the time of presumed viability in law. With modern neonatal developments, the law has reduced this to 24 weeks. Clauses C and D limit terminations to 24 weeks, but the other clauses on death, grave permanent injury to the mother or fetal abnormalities are not time limited. Sometimes ultrasound may only show a fetal abnormality at 26 to 28 weeks or cordocentesis done for karyotyping studies may give results as late as 28 to 29 weeks.

Late termination is repugnant to the woman and to all who have to care for the woman, but it is a logical extension of the law's previous position with more up to date diagnostic tests on the fetus. Such terminations are usually done with prostaglandins and urea.

Menstrual extraction

In some parts of the Western world, notably the USA, a form of self-termination of pregnancy has been used by a few. It derives from menstrual extraction, a technique whereby a small catheter is passed by the woman through her own cervix using a speculum and a mirror. When in the uterine cavity, the catheter is connected to a large syringe and negative pressure removes the endometrium on the first day of menstruation. In theory, this allows the whole menstrual period to be completed in a matter of hours rather than days. However, extraction is rarely complete and so light menstruation goes on. Infection and mild trauma from misplacement of the catheter may occur.

From menstrual extraction has evolved a method of self-termination. If a woman misses a period, then she can pass a catheter a few days after the missed period and apply the same negative pressure. This will disrupt the growing sac and may well extract the fetus. Either way the pregnancy will not proceed and she has performed a self-termination. This is a dangerous practice and has not yet become common in Europe.

Medical termination

The use of antiprogesterone steroids like mifepristone (RU486) has spread from Europe to UK, but not yet to USA because of fears of politicians. It acts by binding to the progesterone receptors allowing transformation. This steroid can be used efficiently at less than 8 weeks of gestation and may avoid the need for surgical uterine evacuation. It is also most useful at 16 to 18 weeks gestation when 200 mg is given 24 hours before prostaglandins ($PGE_{2\alpha}$) and works swiftly.

RU486 can also be injected into ectopic gestational sacs in ectopic pregnancy (Chapter 21) and for post coital emergency contraception.

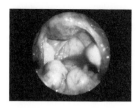

Complications of early pregnancy

Abortion or miscarriage, 249
Causes of spontaneous miscarriage, 249
  Maternal causes, 249
  Fetal causes, 250
  Parental compatibility, 251
  Incidence of spontaneous miscarriage, 251
Clinical features and management, 252

Threatened miscarriage, 252
Inevitable miscarriage, 252
Incomplete miscarriage, 253
Complete miscarriage, 253
Missed abortion, 253
Septic abortion, 254
Criminal abortion, 255

Recurrent abortion, 255
Counselling after miscarriage, 256
Ectopic pregnancy, 257
Hydatidiform mole, 261
  Chorioadenoma destruens (invasive mole), 262
  Chorioncarcinoma, 263

ABORTION OR MISCARRIAGE

An abortion is the expulsion of the products of conception before the 24th week of pregnancy. The word abortion is often considered by our patients to be a procured termination of pregnancy, legal or criminal. Hence, the softer term miscarriage is better used for the spontaneous event. A simple classification is helpful in understanding the various terms used (Fig. 21.1).

CAUSES OF SPONTANEOUS MISCARRIAGE

These may be divided into maternal, fetal and possibly paternal or genetic.

Maternal causes

GENERAL

- Acute febrile illness.
- Septicaemia with infection of the fetus.
- Syphilis (late abortion).
- Severe hypertension and renal disease.

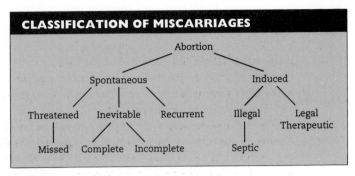

Fig. 21.1 A simple classification of the terms used.

- Diabetes.
- Hypothyroidism.
- Trauma.
- Blow to the abdomen.
- A surgical operation.
- Emotional shock traditionally is a cause, perhaps more in folklore than actuality.

    Drugs like ergot, quinine and lead may be taken to induce abortion. They are not very effective and the risk of poisoning is great.

LOCAL

- Uterine fibroids.
- Congenital malformations.
- Displacement of the uterus.
- Incompetence of the internal os:
    (a) congenital;
    (b) acquired after difficult childbirth, dilatation of the cervix, amputation of the cervix, clumsy attempts to induce abortion.
- Hormone deficiency:
    (a) *progesterone*—the corpus luteum produces progesterone which helps embedding of the embryo. This endocrine function is taken over by the chorion at some time between 80 and 120 days;
    (b) *luteinizing hormone*—polycystic ovary disease has a deficiency of this hormone and a high miscarriage rate.

Fetal causes

- Congenital malformations.
- Genetic abnormalities.

- Faulty implantation.
- Multiple pregnancy.

CONGENITAL AND GENETIC MALFORMATIONS

Examination of the chromosomes in material from spontaneous abortion shows gross abnormalities in over half; the cells may contain 69 or 92 chromosomes (triploidy or tetraploidy).

This is a frequent cause of abortion. In many cases when spontaneous abortion occurs, it is found that the embryo has failed to develop or has been absorbed. In these cases, abortion usually takes place at about eight weeks. Ultrasound shows that the amniotic sac contains no embryo. In other cases, gross malformation of the fetus is shown.

FAULTY IMPLANTATION

The embryo may become implanted in an unfavourable site in the uterus, for example in the isthmus, cervical canal or in the uterine cornu. Most of these cases end in spontaneous abortion, but rarely the cornu may rupture giving a condition which clinically resembles ruptured ectopic pregnancy. A similar picture may follow implantation in a rudimentary horn of the uterus.

Parental compatibility

It has been suggested that sometimes when abortion occurs, the sperm count is low with a high proportion of abnormal forms. This is difficult to prove; it is unlikely that an abnormal sperm would be capable of reaching and fertilizing an oocyte. The possibility of genetic factors must be considered. The existence of lethal genes is well known in the animal kingdom, but their relevance in human genetics is still uncertain.

In normal pregnancies which proceed, some immunological block may occur due to circulating antibodies which protect the fetus against maternal lymphocytes. If by chance the parents are fairly compatible immunologically, there may be a lack of these blocking antibodies produced to protect this developing embryo. Couples with recurrent abortions should be checked so that the parents' blood groups are examined to consider compatibility. If they are compatible, injections of paternal lymphocytes in the woman may generate blocking antibodies and so enhance implantation.

Incidence of spontaneous miscarriage

The frequency of spontaneous abortion depends on definition:

• in clinically diagnosed pregnancies 15 to 20% will miscarry in early pregnancy;

• development of the blastocyst before the next menstrual period (i.e., within 14 days) does not occur in up to 40 to 50% of conceptions.

CLINICAL FEATURES AND MANAGEMENT

Threatened miscarriage

Symptoms
• Uterine bleeding preceded by the symptoms and signs of pregnancy. The bleeding is generally slight.
• Pain is usually absent, but there can be slight backache and a few painful uterine contractions.

Examination
• The breasts may be active.
• The cervix is closed.
• The uterus enlarged corresponding with dates of amenorrhoea.
• There is no pelvic tenderness.

Differential diagnosis
• Missed abortion—the uterus is smaller than would be expected.
• Ectopic pregnancy—pain generally precedes bleeding.
• Dysfunctional uterine bleeding where the signs of pregnancy are absent.
   Ultrasound can show a sac (five weeks), an embryo (six weeks) or the fetal heart beat (seven weeks). hCG can be measured in blood or urine.

TREATMENT
Treatment is usually rest in bed until fresh bleeding has ceased. A sedative such as diazepam 2 mg three times a day may be given.
   After bleeding has ceased, the woman should avoid exertion and travelling, and intercourse should be avoided at least till after the 12th week of pregnancy. Progesterone therapy is ineffective.

Inevitable miscarriage

SYMPTOMS
Bleeding and pain are characteristics; there may be an escape of amniotic fluid.

EXAMINATION

The internal os of the cervix is dilated and products of conception may be felt in the cervical canal. Once this has occurred, miscarriage is inevitable.

TREATMENT

Before 12 weeks gestation, evacuate the uterus under general anaesthesia in an operating theatre.

After 12 weeks, allow miscarriage to take place spontaneously, but be prepared to evacuate the uterus if the abortion is incomplete. If bleeding is severe, Syntometrine should be given, 0.5 mg intramuscularly.

The further into pregnancy, the more probable that the miscarriage is complete.

Incomplete miscarriage

An incomplete miscarriage occurs when some of the products of conception are retained in the uterus. This is usually parts of the placenta which is not fully formed and so is friable; chorionic tissue may be attached to the uterine wall.

The chief symptom is continued bleeding after a period of amenorrhoea. The differential diagnosis is from:

- threatened abortion;
- ectopic pregnancy;
- dysfunctional uterine bleeding.

Ultrasound may help to clarify the diagnosis. The treatment consists of evacuation of the uterus in the operating theatre.

Complete miscarriage

In a complete miscarriage, the products of conception have been passed *per vaginum* and the uterus is empty. There is little bleeding, the uterus is small and the cervix closed or merely patulous in a multiparous woman.

If it is certain that the miscarriage is complete, treatment is rest in bed for a few days. If there is any doubt it is wise to evacuate the uterus.

Missed abortion

The embryo fails to develop or dies in the uterus and the products of conception are retained.

In early missed abortion, there is haemorrhage into the amniotic sac which becomes filled with laminated blood clot and eventually forms a carneous or fleshy mole. The symptoms are at first those of pregnancy, but these disappear, the breasts become soft and a small dark brown vaginal discharge may appear. The cervix is closed and the uterus smaller than would be expected had pregnancy continued. The pregnancy test becomes negative in seven to ten days.

Differential diagnosis:

- tubal mole;
- an incomplete miscarriage;
- a complete miscarriage.

Ultrasound will confirm the diagnosis.

TREATMENT

Evacuate the uterus if it is no more than 12 weeks' size. Later emptying of the uterus may be induced using prostaglandin in the form of vaginal pessaries or vaginal gel. There is a remote risk of afibrinogenaemia in late cases of missed abortion.

Septic abortion

Infection of the uterine cavity following an abortion leads to septic abortion. It can occur after spontaneous abortion, but most cases result from criminal interference with non-sterile instruments.

Spreading infection leads rapidly to salpingitis, pelvic peritonitis, pelvic cellulitis, septicaemia and pyaemia. Infection with *tetanus* will give the typical features of the disease and can be fatal. Infection with *Clostridium welchii* is not uncommon in criminal abortions; the picture is that of severe infection with shock and tachycardia. Such cases need prompt and efficient treatment preferably in an intensive care unit.

The diagnosis of septic abortion is made on a history of abortion, often criminal, and of the signs of pelvic infection and septicaemia. There is fever, pelvic pain and tenderness with foul discharge from the uterus and bleeding. A neutrophil leucocytosis is found on the blood count and the haemoglobin level may be reduced.

TREATMENT

- Admission to hospital.
- Swabs should be taken for cultures from the cervix and blood culture taken in seriously ill patients.
- Adequate doses of antibiotics should start at once; a combination of amoxycillin, clindamycin and metronidazole may be used initially. A change of antibiotic may be needed when the cultures and sensitivities become available.
- Gas gangrene serum is no longer used, as modern antibiotics are more effective.

- Full intravenous supportive measures and steroids may be needed.

If the products of conception are retained, the uterus should be evacuated. This should only be done at once if there is severe bleeding, otherwise it is preferable to wait to allow the antibiotics to take effect.

Criminal abortion

Under the Offences against the Person Act 1861, any attempt to procure abortion by the woman herself or by another person is a felony, irrespective of whether she is in fact pregnant. The position of termination of pregnancy under the Abortion Act is considered in Chapter 20.

Abortion may be procured by:
- drugs;
- instruments passed into the uterus;
- foreign bodies such as slippery elm bark introduced into the cervix;
- injections of soap pastes or douching with soap or antiseptic solutions.

Criminal abortion is dangerous:
- drugs may cause poisoning;
- infection can easily be introduced;
- risk of severe haemorrhage can occur;
- embolism with air or soap solution.

The doctor called to deal with a woman who had a criminal abortion is bound to respect her confidence. He or she should not inform the police or any other person unless the woman dies or appears likely to do so, when a dying declaration should be obtained. Deaths must be reported to the coroner.

Recurrent abortion

Three consecutive spontaneous abortions constitutes habitual abortion. It may be primary where the woman is borne no viable child, or secondary. The most important causes are:
- Maternal:
  (a) incompetence of the cervix;
      trauma of the cervix;
      previous difficult labour;
      repeated dilatation of the cervix;
      operations of the cervix;
  (b) congenital malformation of the uterus;
  (c) antinuclear antibodies;
  (d) systemic lupus erythematosis.
- Fetal:
  a series of blighted embryos, usually genetic in origin.

MANAGEMENT

This depends on the time in pregnancy when it occurs. If early in pregnancy, the patient should rest, especially when menstruation is due. She is wise to abstain from exertion, intercourse and travelling until after the 14th week. The pregnancy should be monitored by ultrasound to ensure that the fetus is present and developing normally. Late recurrent abortion after the 12th week is often due to incompetence of the cervix which may require suturing prophylactically.

INVESTIGATIONS

Between pregnancies hysterosalpinography showing an incompetent internal os. This may also reveal a congenital malformation of the uterus.

In pregnancy, ultrasound is sometimes helpful in showing the same deficiency.

TREATMENT

During pregnancy a cervical suture may be inserted, preferably at about the 14th week of pregnancy. The cervix is encircled by a ribbon of non-absorbable material (Fig. 21.2). The suture remains in place until the 38th week of pregnancy unless the woman aborts or goes into preterm labour, in which case it must be removed at once or the cervix may tear. If the membranes rupture prematurely, it is also wise to remove the suture to prevent ascending infection.

The operation is reserved for those cases where incompetence of the cervix is proved or strongly presumed on the previous history. A deeply torn cervix may require repair by trachelorrhaphy between pregnancies.

Counselling after miscarriage

Counselling is often needed for the woman who has undergone a spontaneous miscarriage and for her partner. A spontaneous miscarriage may lead to bereavement even though the event is early in pregnancy and the woman may not identify it with a baby. It is important that the woman and her partner receive an explanation of what happened and of the possible cause of the miscarriage if it is known. If there is a treatable cause, such as uterine fibroids, treatment should be planned as soon as possible though the operation itself may be best postponed for about three months.

The couple anxious to have a baby will often ask how soon they should try for another pregnancy. In most normal cases, where no serious cause is identified, there is no reason why they should not immediately, that is, as soon as the woman has had a normal period or

CERVICAL CIRCLAGE

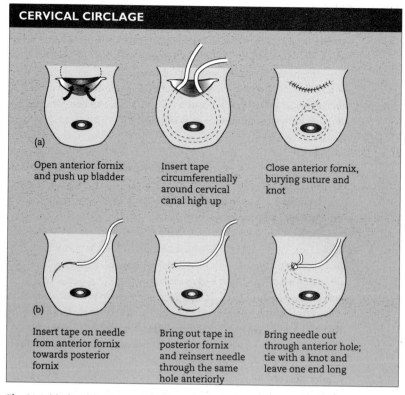

(a)

Open anterior fornix and push up bladder

Insert tape circumferentially around cervical canal high up

Close anterior fornix, burying suture and knot

(b)

Insert tape on needle from anterior fornix towards posterior fornix

Bring out tape in posterior fornix and reinsert needle through the same hole anteriorly

Bring needle out through anterior hole; tie with a knot and leave one end long

Fig. 21.2 (a) The Shirodkar and (b) Macdonald sutures.

two. Commonly given advice to wait three to six months has no logical basis.

ECTOPIC PREGNANCY

Ectopic pregnancy is one outside the uterine cavity; the commonest site is the fallopian tube. Ectopic pregnancy may also occur, although rarely, in:

- uterine cornu;
- the ovary;
- the cervix;
- the abdominal cavity;
- the broad ligament.

For practical purposes, ectopic pregnancy will be considered as tubal pregnancy.

INCIDENCE

Estimates of the incidence of tubal pregnancy vary. In England it is about one in every 250 to 300 pregnancies. In other countries, especially in those with large Negro populations, it may be as high as 1% because of the higher prevalence of chronic tubal disease.

CAUSES

The ovum is usually fertilized in the fallopian tube and reaches the uterus in about five days. Within a day or so of this, the trophoblast is sufficiently developed for implantation. Anything which delays the passage of the fertilized ovum to the uterus can result in tubal pregnancy.

Salpingitis is the commonest predisposing cause. This may not be so severe as to cause complete closing of the tube, but it may destroy tubal cilia or kink or narrow the tube. *Tuberculous salpingitis* is an important but rare cause, for it damages the tube but often leaves it patent.

Congenital malformation of the tube may lead to crypts and diverticula providing sites for ectopic implantation.

Contra-lateral implantation is where the fertilized ovum may come from one ovary, but may be carried into the opposite tube. Its passage to the uterus thus takes longer than usual and trophoblast may so develop that implantation takes place in the tube. In such cases the tubal pregnancy should be on one side and the corpus luteum of the pregnancy in the opposite ovary.

PATHOLOGY

The embryo does not grow beyond a certain size in the tube. The trophoblast gradually invades and erodes the tubal wall which, unlike the endometrium, is not prepared for implantation. Blood vessels are damaged and eventually bleeding takes place.

A tubal pregnancy may terminate in a number of ways.

• *Absorption*—in a few cases it is possible that absorption of a very early tubal pregnancy occurs.

• *Tubal mole*—this is the commonest termination. The embryo dies in the tube, with a small amount of bleeding, and is partly absorbed. This is a similar condition to the carneous mole of missed abortion in the uterus.

• *Pelvic haematocoele*—bleeding is more extensive and a collection of blood forms in the pelvic cavity. This is often associated with tubal abortion; part or all of the products of conception being expelled from the tube into the peritoneal cavity.

• *Tubal rupture*—this is the most dramatic and best known termination of a tubal pregnancy, though in fact less common than tubal mole or tubal abortion. There is acute intra-peritoneal haemorrhage from erosion of an artery. The pregnancy is often implanted in the narrower isthmus of the tube.

• *Secondary abdominal pregnancy*—this is the rarest outcome of all. The embryo is expelled complete from the tube and acquires a secondary attachment in the peritoneal cavity. It can occasionally go on to full term abdominal pregnancy. Many cases of normal children delivered from the peritoneal cavity have been reported, but others are born with gross deformities or die before delivery. When a fetus dies in the abdominal cavity, a lithopaedion is formed.

CLINICAL FEATURES

The classical picture of ectopic pregnancy includes a number of symptoms.

• *Amenorrhoea*—this is usually four to eight weeks' duration, but may present before amenorrhoea is noticed.

• *Pain*—typically cramp-like, colicky and often unilateral due to spasm of the tubal muscle. There may be referred pain to shoulder.

• *Vaginal bleeding*—while a pregnancy is implanting in the tube, the uterine endometrium is converted into decidua. When the embryo dies in the tube, the decidua in the uterus separates. The bleeding is usually scanty, less than a normal period and dark brown in colour.

• *Faintness* or even *shock* with an acute rupture.

An undisturbed ectopic pregnancy may have the following:

• slight activity of the breasts;

• slight tenderness over one side of the uterus.

On bimanual examination, the uterus is slightly enlarged and the cervix is soft. There may be dark blood oozing from the external os. The pregnant tube may be palpable or more likely there will be a tenderness to one side of the uterus.

A tubal mole gives a similar clinical picture but the mole is generally easily palpable as a slightly tender swelling in the lateral fornix.

A *pelvic haematocoele* often has a fibrin layer on its surface, forming light adhesions to the bowel. It presents with abdominal and pelvic pain.

An abdominal mass may be palpable. On bimanual examination, the haematocoele is felt as a diffuse boggy swelling. It is of any size, it displaces the uterus to the opposite side of the pelvis. It must be distinguished from a retroverted gravid uterus, from torsion or haemorrhage into an ovarian cyst, from pyosalpinx, from degenerating fibroid or carcinoma of the ovary.

INVESTIGATIONS

Ultrasound is helpful. While it usually cannot show the embryo or its sac in the tube because gestation may not be far enough advanced, ultrasound findings may be:

- an empty uterus with thickened decidua;
- fluid (blood) in the pouch of Douglas;
- a multi-echo mass in the region of the tube.

Laparoscopy is the ultimate investigation to make the diagnosis with direct vision.

Acute rupture presents as an abdominal catastrophe. The patient collapses with severe abdominal pain, pallor, shock, rapid pulse and hypotension. Blood may track up under the diaphragm giving shoulder pain. The abdomen is slightly distended, tender and rigid. On vaginal examination, the uterus is soft and may be enlarged with a tender tubal mass apart from it; usually the tube cannot be palpated because of the extreme tenderness.

DIFFERENTIAL DIAGNOSIS

The diagnosis is from any other abdominal catastrophe such as rupture of a viscus or acute peritonitis. The clinical picture is so typical that in most cases diagnosis presents no difficulty. Other diagnoses which may confuse are:

- incomplete abortion;
- bleeding with an ovarian cyst;
- pelvic appendicitis;
- acute salpingitis.

TREATMENT

The treatment of tubal pregnancy is laparoscopy or laparotomy with removal of the pregnancy and sometimes the affected tube. If the tube is patent and not seriously damaged, it may be possible to conserve it and thus leave the woman with a chance of conception later in life.

Laparoscopy techniques now exist to:

- kill the embryo with a direct injection of methotrexate or mifepristone allowing absorption so requiring no surgery on the tube;
- incise over the swollen tube over the ectopic pregnancy, aspirate the embryo, achieve haemostasis and resuture the tube.

In a case of severe haemorrhage, the patient must be taken immediately to the operating theatre. Little time should be wasted in attempting resuscitation; this may prove useless and will only increase bleeding. An intravenous drip should be set up and a blood transfusion given as soon as possible. It is sometimes possible to collect the extravasated blood from the peritoneal cavity with a cellsaver and return it to the circulation.

In most cases the affected tube should be removed; an exception may be made if the woman desires children and the other tube is already missing or seriously diseased. The disadvantage of conservation is the distinct risk of recurrence of ectopic pregnancy.

Tubal pregnancy and normal intrauterine pregnancy may occur simultaneously in very rare circumstances.

HYDATIDIFORM MOLE

Hydatidiform mole is a benign tumour of both parts of the chorion: the cytotrophoblast and the syncytiotrophoblast may be found in varying proportions. The villi undergo cystic or hydropic degeneration and a certain amount of bleeding almost always occurs.

Hydatidiform moles vary greatly in their rate of growth, in the amount of chorionic gonadotrophin produced and in the amount of invasion of the uterine wall.

Only rarely can a fetus be found, but hydatidiform degeneration may occur in the placenta in cases of abortion. The birth of a living fetus with a hydatidiform mole has been described.

INCIDENCE

In the UK one in 2500 pregnancies. The condition appears to be much commoner in women in the Far East than elsewhere in the world; malignant change also appears to be commoner in these parts.

CLINICAL FEATURES

The typical clinical features are amenorrhoea followed by continuous or intermittent vaginal bleeding. The other symptoms of pregnancy occur, often exaggerated; vomiting may be severe and pre-eclampsia may develop. The uterus is often larger than the dates would suggest and feels very soft and boggy. Theca lutein cysts may develop in the ovaries.

Part of the mole may be passed spontaneously and this is diagnostic of the condition.

INVESTIGATIONS

Chorionic gonadotrophin excretion in urine is often greater than other pregnancies, while levels of 40000 to 60000 iu/l are common, concentrations of over 1000000 iu/l are generally diagnostic of a mole. No fetus can be demonstrated on X-ray.

Ultrasonic examination is reliable in showing the absence of a fetus and the characteristic picture of foam or soap bubbles (bright sunlight shining through the washing-up water).

TREATMENT

The uterus must be emptied completely in all cases. If there seems to be spontaneous evacuation, the uterus must still be carefully aspirated and curetted.

An intact mole may be dealt with by suction evacuation of the mole, then curetting the cavity gently to ensure as far as possible that the mole has been removed. Intravenous syntometrine must be given to minimize bleeding. The use of suction to evacuate the uterus is safest and carries less risk of perforation than curettage. Dangers include:

- haemorrhage which can be profuse;
- sepsis;
- perforation of the uterus;
- air embolism;
- incomplete evacuation of the uterus.

A second aspiration or curettage may be needed two to four weeks later to be sure that the mole has been completely removed.

Hysterotomy is now rarely performed but it may be wise to offer a hysterectomy with the mole *in situ* for women who do not desire further children or in cases of intra-peritoneal haemorrhage with a perforating mole.

FOLLOW-UP

The woman should be followed-up by regular estimations of beta sub-units of hCG for at least a year and should avoid pregnancy.

Tests should be carried out monthly for the first six months and after that every two months. Persistence of hCG after one month may suggest incomplete evacuation of the uterus or malignant change. This would indicate chemotherapeutic treatment with actinomycin D or metholtrexate as a prophylaxis against choriocarcinoma. Another normal pregnancy may cause difficulty in diagnosis if a previously low hCG level rises.

During the period of follow-up, the woman should not take the contraceptive pill; barrier methods of contraception should be used.

Chorioadenoma destruens (invasive mole)

In some cases of hydatidiform mole, there may be great trophoblastic activity with penetration of the uterine wall. There may be a simple invasive mole which causes the uterine enlargement and bleeding with a positive pregnancy test; these may require hysterectomy. In other cases trophoblast penetrates to the peritoneum or into the parametrium and leads to internal haemorrhage. The level of hCG is high. These cases require urgent hysterectomy.

Chorioncarcinoma

This malignant tumour invades the uterine wall and metastasizes widely through the blood-stream. Rarely primary tumours are found in the ovary or testis as a form of teratoma.

It is fortunately an unusual tumour; about 40% follow hydatidiform mole, 37% follow abortion and 23% pregnancy at term. Conversely, a hydatidiform mole may go on to choriocarcinoma in 4 to 5% of women compared with 1 per 50 000 after normal pregnancy.

CLINICAL FEATURES

Uterine bleeding is the commonest symptom. Secondaries may appear rapidly and are most often found in the lungs, the uterus and the vagina, but they can involve the liver and the central nervous system. The levels of hCG are very high often above 100 000 iu/l.

Chorioncarcinoma is sensitive to cytotoxic drugs and is now curable in the majority of patients. Those with low grade disease treated with methotrexate can retain their fertility and have further successful pregnancies. Assay of hCG in serum or urine is used as a tumour marker and reduction in its levels is a test of cure.

Chemotherapy is best given in units which specialize in its use and various combinations of drugs are given; methotrexate is the first line of attack and may be combined with vincristine, cyclophosphamide and actinomycin D.

With modern treatment, hysterectomy is now rarely indicated except with massive tumours causing severe bleeding and when the response to chemotherapy is poor.

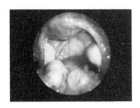

CHAPTER 22

The acute abdomen in gynaecology

Pain, 265
Shock, 266
Nausea and vomiting, 266
Distension, 267
Diagnosis, 267
Conditions to be
    considered, 269
Out of pregnancy, 269
    Vaginal trauma, 269
    Uterine fibroids, 269

Salpingitis, 270
Pyosalpinx, 271
Torsion of the fallopian
    tube, 271
Ovarian tumour, 271
Endometriosis, 272
In pregnancy, 272
Abortion, 272
Retroverted uterus, 272

Red degeneration of
    fibroid, 273
Ectopic pregnancy, 273
Round ligament stretch,
    274
Pyelonephritis, 274
Appendicitis, 274
Rectus haematoma, 275
Bowel problems, 275

Many diseases causing acute lower abdominal symptoms are gynaecological in origin. The general surgeon and gynaecologist must both be trained to recognize and deal with conditions of the lower abdomen. When available, consultation will take place but delay and mortality are linked and acute abdominal conditions do not leave time for leisurely consultations. If the condition is obviously gynaecological in origin, it is best dealt with by gynaecologists as they are more used to conservation of genital tract tissue, particularly the ovaries.

Acute intra-abdominal emergencies present with pain, shock, vomiting or abdominal distension. The first of these is the most common in gynaecological conditions.

PAIN

Pain in pelvic organs may arise from:
- inside the organ with irritation of its lining or stretch of its walls;
- stretch of the visceral peritoneum over the organ;
- involvement of the parietal peritoneum in proximity.

    For example, an ectopic pregnancy can cause pain from:
- damage to the muscle of the oviduct by trophoblast invasion and bleeding;
- stretch of the peritoneum of the broad ligament over the fallopian tube at the site of the pregnancy;

- blood spilt onto the peritoneum by the rupture of the tube (acute) or trickling from the outer end of the tube (chronic).

The first two origins of stimulae are mediated by the autonomic nervous system with poor localization; hence non-specific pain in the hypergastrium results.

The parietal peritoneum is innervated by the somatic nervous system and localization may be more specific. The peritoneum of the pouch of Douglas has a poor nerve supply and is often undemonstrative. Since this is the area in which the tubes and ovaries spend much of their time, it makes pain localization in the abdominal wall difficult in pelvic acute abdominal conditions in the earlier stages, but signs are easier to detect on pelvic and rectal examination.

SHOCK

A sudden deterioration in a woman's vital state may be characterized by:
- a rise followed by a fall in pulse rate;
- a fall in arterial blood pressure;
- pallor;
- faintness and later unconsciousness.

This may be due to either:
- true hypovolaemia e.g., a ruptured ectopic pregnancy with two litres of blood in the peritoneal cavity;
- relative hypovolaemia, e.g., excess of autonomic stimulation after peritoneal irritation with blood or a sudden release of pus.

Pallor, sweating, agitation and restlessness are traditional indications of shock, of which pallor is the most important for prognosis in the gynaecological field. Fainting and unconsciousness come later in shock and may be considered as signs of more extensive involvement.

NAUSEA AND VOMITING

These happen early in acute gynaecological conditions due to a number of causes.
- Stimulation of a large number of nerve endings of the peritoneum overlying an affected pelvic organ.
- The direct action of toxins on the central nervous system from infective organisms. Pelvic inflammation often becomes localized early and toxins are released intermittently into the general blood stream as pressure rises.
- Vomiting is a common accompaniment of early pregnancy. Many gynaecological conditions happen in early gestation so vomiting might be

nothing to do with the acute condition in the pelvis but more to the hCG produced by the pregnancy trophoblast.

DISTENSION

Distension is unusual in gynaecological conditions but common in alimentary tract ones, particularly those of the large bowel. In consequence, if distension is present, it is probably due to an associated bowel problem following a gynaecological one.

DIAGNOSIS

The triad of history, examination and investigations applies here as anywhere else in medicine. This section is to be read in conjunction with the account of gynaecological diagnosis making in Chapter 1.

HISTORY

Women in severe acute abdominal pain do not like having long histories taken. Hence, the questions must be tailored to the situation.

Pain
- Characteristics of the pain site, time and nature.
- Relationship of pain to various body functions, e.g., vaginal bleeding or micturition.
- Past gynaecological or obstetrical events.
- Menstrual history i.e., details of last menstrual period.
- Symptoms of a possible pregnancy, e.g., breast changes and the woman's own impressions.

EXAMINATION

A general examination must cover a number of points.
- Paleness (conjunctival assessment).
- Pulse rate.
- Arterial blood pressure.
- Temperature.
- Abdominal examination helps to localize pelvic causes.
- *Observation* will show old scars and the degree of distention; the site of the pain can be elicited from the woman at this point.
- *Gentle palpation* of the abdomen leading to the lower pelvic zones may help localization further.
- *Firmer examination* – if tenderness allows, this will reveal guarding or any rebound tenderness.

• Many pelvic acute abdominal conditions do not have specific localizing signs in the abdomen and so, therefore, any opinion should await the performing of a bimanual vaginal examination.

• The *bimanual vaginal assessment* during which signs are gathered not just by the fingers in the vagina but those on the abdominal wall as well. When done properly in a thin patient, in effect a medical laparotomy of the pelvis can be easily and gently performed.

Tenderness from a pelvic organ will obviously limit the thoroughness of a vaginal examination for the woman will guard if there is pain on moving the cervix. Such cervical excitation is not necessarily a sign of an ectopic pregnancy for there may be some other problem in the pouch of Douglas irritating the peritoneum overlying the uterus or its ligaments.

• *Rectal examination* may be needed but usually one can assess acute pouch of Douglas problems at a vaginal assessment. If structural changes are sought in the back of the pelvic cavity, the rectal examination is useful — e.g., endometriotic lesions on the utero-sacral ligaments.

Other special examinations may involve asking the woman to stand and stamp her foot. The shock wave passing up through the bones of the tibia and femur will arrive at the femoral head which is only a few millimetres from the pelvic cavity through the acetabular cup. Involvement of the peritoneum may often produce pain on this simple sign. Straight leg extension test sometimes demonstrates irritation over the psoas muscle. Flexion with thigh rotation test may also give some clues of pelvic inflammation.

INVESTIGATIONS

There are a few investigations that help.

• Haemoglobin to check on chronic bleeding.
• Differential white cell count to assess inflammation.
• Urine cells and organisms to diagnose urinary infection.
• hCG levels to check for pregnancy.
• High vaginal swab to test for genital tract infection.
• X-rays may be used to check for bowel obstruction.
• Ultrasound is extremely useful to check the pelvic organs, particularly with a vaginal probe. Then the transmitter and receiver are within a centimetre or two of the affected organs.

The vaginal ultrasound examination gives far more precise images of pelvic organs and tissues.

• Changes in ovarian morphology and size:
    (a) cysts;
    (b) polycystic ovary syndrome;
    (c) irregular masses.
• Fallopian tube:

(a) occasionally a swollen tube from a pyo- or hydrosalpinx is identified;

(b) ectopic pregnancies usually will not be seen *per se* (Chapter 21).

• Uterine size can be detected:

(a) the thickness of the endometrium is shown;

(b) the presence of a pregnancy sac can be detected as early as five weeks, embryonic parts by six weeks and fetal heart beats by seven weeks from the last menstrual period.

• Fibroids of the uterus.

• Fluid in the pouch of Douglas can often be detected in as low a volume as 7 ml. This might indicate blood loss from an ectopic pregnancy.

Often a combination of ultrasound with other tests is helpful. For example, in the UK now, many unruptured ectopic pregnancies are diagnosed in symptomatic women who have an empty uterus but a thickened endometrium and fluid in the pouch of Douglas at ultrasound in the presence of raised urinary hCG levels.

CONDITIONS TO BE CONSIDERED

We diagnose what we are thinking of and it is helpful to have a check list (Box 22.1). The majority of these conditions are dealt with elsewhere in this book. The aspects that are important in diagnosis of an acute abdominal emergency only are considered here.

OUT OF PREGNANCY

Vaginal trauma

Intercourse occurring forcibly or after a long interval of abstinence can cause damage to the vaginal tube.

• Lower end – usually obvious but may be labial or fourchette.

• Upper end – vaginal guarding to prevent the easy passage of the speculum. Hence, hard to see.

• Haematoma – para-vaginal or para-cervical haematoma.

The obvious point needed in the history may not be volunteered readily. Treatment is by vaginal repair under anaesthesia.

Uterine fibroids

Usually fibroids enlarge slowly. Mostly they cause no pain having their effect through menstrual upset. Pain implies a complication such as torsion which may happen with a pedunculated fibroid or degeneration

PELVIC DISEASES

	Organ	Condition
Non pregnant		
	Vagina	Trauma
	Uterus	Fibroid
		Torsion
		Degeneration
	Fallopian tubes	Salpingitis
		Pylosalpinx
		Torsion
	Ovaries	Tumours
		Simple cyst
		Torsion
		Bleeding
		Rupture
	Peritoneum	Endometriosis
Early pregnancy		
	Uterus	Abortion
		Impacted retroversion
		Red degeneration of fibroids
	Fallopian tubes	Ectopic pregnancy
		Torsion
	Ligaments	Round ligament
		Stretch
	Extra pelvic	Vomiting in pregnancy
		Pyelonephritis
		Appendicitis
		Rectus haematoma

Box 22.1 Pelvic diseases presenting as acute abdominal emergencies.

with a decreased blood supply. The former is fairly sudden while the latter is rather slow. Local tenderness over a previously diagnosed fibroid may be present.

Treatment is usually supportive until the acute phase settles and then surgical after an interval.

Salpingitis

Infection of fallopian tubes rarely stops at that. It usually becomes a parametritis, an oophoritis, and may even go to pelvic peritonitis. The woman looks ill. She is vomiting, has a high temperature and often rigors. There is usually bilateral tenderness and guarding, sometimes with distention. Slight movement of the cervix produces pain and there may be a purulent vaginal discharge.

Treatment is conservative with bedrest, local heat and antibiotics.

This diagnosis can only be made definitively by laparoscopy which shows a red, inflamed pair of tubes.

Pyosalpinx

Usually the pain is chronic but occasionally one pus tube will burst and the woman presents with an acute abdomen. Laparoscopy will confirm the condition if there are not too many obscuring adhesions.

If diagnosed, a pyosalpinx is usually best treated conservatively with possible interval surgery on the fallopian tube. At the time of first diagnosis the area is usually oedematous, bound down and would be difficult to remove leaving much bleeding from raw areas.

Torsion of the fallopian tube

This rare complication usually occurs in association with torsion of the ovary. The tube is long and on a long mesosalpinx.

The diagnosis is commonly not made until the abdomen is opened and a laparoscopy usually gives confusing findings. The torted part of the fallopian tube might need excision if it is no longer viable. Occasionally unwinding may be possible and if viable gonadal tissue should be preserved. Fixation to the pelvic side wall may prevent recurrence.

Ovarian tumour

An ovarian tumour is often cystic and may increase in size rapidly. It may undergo:
- torsion with the ovary;
- a cyst which may rupture;
- haemorrhage occurring into the lumen of a cyst.

There is peritoneal irritation leading to a degree of shock and a tendency to abdominal muscle guarding.

After resuscitation, a laparoscopy is usually required. In skilled hands, minimal access surgery through a laparoscope can deal with an obviously simple ovarian cyst, which has either undergone torsion or has bled. If there is doubt about whether the tumour is malignant, many surgeons prefer to open the abdomen at laparotomy to perform a formal resection. Some skilled and adventurous laparoscope-adept gynaecologists are starting to deal with this by minimal access surgery, enclosing the tumour in a plastic bag to ensure no spill of malignant cells. They then divide it from the other pelvic organs and remove it through an incision in the pouch of Douglas.

Endometriosis

This is usually a more chronic condition producing lower abdominal pain, particularly at the time of intercourse or menstruation along with heavy periods. However, blood cysts can accumulate and may suddenly cause pain by stretch or rupture.

Laparoscopy is required to make the diagnosis; after suction and lavage, treatment is with hormones or anti-hormones. Very rarely is surgery needed. Laser may be used with a laparoscope to dispose of smaller lesions while surgical removal of larger blood cysts is more usual.

IN PREGNANCY

Abortion

Pregnancies which stop before 24 weeks usually are accompanied by pain. Typically these are cramping hypogastric pains associated with vaginal bleeding, although this is not a pattern that is always seen. Usually pain implies that the miscarriage process has gone from threatened to inevitable but the woman may present with lower abdominal pain, backache and vomiting. She may be toxic and the lower abdomen tender with possible rebound tenderness. She may not want to give a full history of the miscarriage and its preceding intercourse so diagnostic problems can arise.

These can be elucidated by pelvic examination which usually shows the cervix to be open with blood coming through it. If the miscarriage is incomplete, a curettage will usually be needed. If there is sepsis the woman will probably have a septic endometritis with salpo-oophoritis and, at a later stage, pelvic cellulitis. Treatment is conservative with antibiotics and bedrest to prevent the spread of sepsis and the sequelae toxic shock (see Chapter 20).

Retroverted uterus

A tipped back uterus is common and when the woman becomes pregnant, it usually rises up in the pelvis at about 12 weeks of gestation. If, however, it is incarcerated by old adhesions, the uterus may dislocate the bladder upwards and stretch the urethra. This can produce acute pain and retention of urine. The situation is usually sorted out by bimanual examination.

Treatment is usually by continuous drainage of the bladder for a few days so the uterus rights itself or intrauterine growth goes on by anterior sacculation of the uterine wall.

Red degeneration of fibroid

Red degeneration is common in early pregnancy usually coming between 12 and 20 weeks of gestation. There is sudden tenderness of a mass in the lower abdomen associated with the uterus. As blood spreads in the fibroid, it stuffs it with extracellular red cells.

If diagnosed with confidence, the best treatment is analgesia and correction of shock or any dehydration. If there is doubt, a laparotomy would be wise. If surgeons then see the oedematous dark red fibroid they would do well to leave it and not attempt a myomectomy during the pregnancy.

Ectopic pregnancy

Whilst this applies to all pregnancies outside the cavity of the uterus, those in the fallopian tube are by far the commonest. They often present as a mild lower abdominal pain with backache which accompanies the unruptured leaking ectopic with a dribble of blood from the fallopian tube.

When the tubal ectopic pregnancy ruptures releasing up to one or two litres of blood into the peritoneal cavity, an acute abdomen presents. The woman can be in shock, the degree according to the blood loss and irritation of the peritoneum. The abdomen is rigid and often no signs can be gathered because of spasm of the rectus muscles. Vaginal examination is extremely tender particularly around the cervix.

Severe shock may need correction but surgery often cannot await full resuscitation. Hence treatment is immediate surgical operation to achieve haemostasis whilst shock correction is proceeding. A laparoscopy under general anaesthesia is only a useful investigation if there is doubt. It the patient is ill, many surgeons would proceed straight to a laparotomy and remove the tube.

If the woman is less shocked, minimally invasive surgery through the laparoscope allows the tube or the ectopic pregnancy to be removed and the bleeding stopped. The full management of an ectopic pregnancy is considered in Chapter 21.

Round ligament stretch

As the uterus rises in the abdomen, it pulls on the surrounding ligaments like an inflating hot-air balloon stretching its guy ropes. The tension on the ligaments becomes too much and a haematoma follows.

The woman has sudden lower abdominal pain which is localized over the haematoma and can often be followed along the course of the ligament as it passes down to the pubic tubercle where there is acute, referred tenderness.

Treatment, if made with confidence is conservative—bedrest, local warmth and anaesthesia.

Pyelonephritis

Urinary infection is common in pregnancy and is dealt with in detail in the companion volume, *Lecture Notes on Obstetrics*, sixth edition.

The woman presents with ill defined abdominal pain, pyrexia and shivering. The diagnosis differs from an acute abdominal problem for the pain is often round the side in the loin and tenderness is then high up in the costal angles.

Examination of the urine for pus cells and organisms reveals the diagnosis. Treatment is conservative with bedrest, fluids, and appropriate antibiotics.

Very rarely a ureteric stone may present in pregnancy. If this sticks in the ureter, it causes pain by stretch of the dammed-back urine behind it. Pethidine is helpful both for its analgesia properties and because it is an antispasmodic.

Appendicitis

This occurs equally commonly in early pregnancy as during any other nine months of a young woman's life. It is a young person's disease.

Diagnosis can be difficult for the appendix rises up from its usual position in the right iliac fossa. The typical history of peri-umbilical pain moving to the right iliac fossa may not be given in pregnancy; the signs are confusing as the caecum with its attached appendix is pushed up the right paracolic gutter by the enlarging uterus. Remembering this, the examiner must seek the point of maximum tenderness higher in the abdomen.

Treatment should be by surgery and the surgeon in later pregnancy would do well to mark the site of maximum tenderness before the anaesthetic and incise there rather than over McBurney's point.

There used to be a higher mortality of appendicitis in pregnancy because of the reluctance of people to operate for fear of miscarriage.

However, it must be realized that a progressing appendicitis carries a much higher risk to the fetus and mother than the problems of carrying out a surgical procedure under controlled anaesthesia.

Rectus haematoma

The deep epigastric arteries with their concomitant epigastric veins are stretched by the growing uterus and occasionally, after a severe attack of coughing, one of these veins under tension may rupture. This leads to a haematoma that is very difficult to diagnose. If seen early, the pain is localized under one segment of one rectus muscle but after a few hours this sign spreads. If seen very late, there may be anaemia due to loss of blood from the circulation.

If diagnosed competently, surgical treatment is not needed. Occasionally, a laparotomy is performed and the diagnosis becomes obvious when the rectus muscles are separated before opening the peritoneum. Usually it is too late to ligate any of the veins. The operator need proceed no further.

Bowel problems

Should a gynaecologist open the abdomen and find a bowel or peritoneal problem, he would be wise to consult with a surgical colleague urgently. Although gynaecologists may have been trained once to do general surgery they do not practise such operations daily. Combined surgical and gynaecological operating would probably be better for the woman.

CHAPTER 23

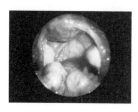

Gynaecological surgery

Vaginal and vulval
operations, 277
Dilatation and curettage
(D&C), 277
Other vaginal operations,
278
Vulvectomy, 279
Laparoscopy, 279
Colpoperineorrhaphy,
280

Vaginal hysterectomy,
280
Abdominal operations, 281
Hysterectomy, 281
Myomectomy, 282
Ventrosuspension, 282
Operations on the fallopian
tubes, 283
Salpingectomy, 283
Other operations, 283

Operations on the ovaries,
283
Radical operations, 284
Appendicectomy, 284
Pre-operative preparation,
284
Clinical examination, 285
Preparation, 285
Post-operative care, 287
Post-operative
complications, 287

All gynaecological operations are best learnt in the operating theatre, preferably acting as a scrubbed assistant.

VAGINAL AND VULVAL OPERATIONS

Dilatation and curettage (D&C)

This is the most frequently performed gynaecological operation and a brief account will be given.

- The patient is anaesthetized and placed in the lithotomy position.
- The external genitalia and vagina are cleaned with an antiseptic solution. If diathermy is to be used, solutions in spirit must not be used.
- A bimanual examination is performed to determine the size and position of the uterus.
- If the bladder is filled, it is emptied with a catheter.
- A weighted speculum is inserted into the vagina and the cervix is grasped with a volsellum.
- A sound is gently passed into the uterus to measure the uterine cavity.
- The cervix is gently dilated with graduated metal dilators to about 8 mm.
- If a hysteroscope is to be used, it is inserted at this point.
- The uterine cavity is explored with sponge forceps to remove any

polypi and is curetted systematically; any irregularity such as submucous fibroid is noted.

• The curettings are labelled and sent to the laboratory for histological examination.

• In the rare case where tuberculosis is suspected, culture of the curettings may be undertaken.

Listed below are the indications for dilatation and curettage.

DIAGNOSTIC

• Dysfunctional bleeding.
• Sterility.
• Amenorrhoea.
• Oligomenorrhoea.
• Malignant disease of the uterus.

THERAPEUTIC

• To remove the retained products of conception following abortion.
• To perform therapeutic or legal termination of pregnancy.
• The removal of polypi and small submucous fibroids.
• The removal of an intrauterine device.
• To drain a pyometra or haematometra.
• As part of the application of caesium or other forms of local radiotherapy.

A D&C may be combined with minor operations of the cervix including:
• cauterization;
• biopsy;
• conization;
• laser treatment.

CONTRA-INDICATIONS

• Pregnancy.
• Sepsis of the vagina or cervix.

Other vaginal operations

• Colpotomy—the vagina is incised through the posterior fornix to open the peritoneum to drain a pelvic abscess.
• Hymenectomy may be required if a rigid hymen makes coitus impossible.
• Perineotomy—the perineal body is divided and the introitus sutured to result in plastic enlargement.
• An artificial vagina may be constructed by flaps of skin or by the

insertion of a mould covered with a skin graft from the thigh into a cavity made between the vagina and the rectum.

• Warts may be removed with diathermy and other benign tumours excised. Cysts and abscesses of *Bartholin's gland* are marsupialized (Fig. 23.1).

• An urethral caruncle may be treated by diathermic excision. Prolapse of the urethral mucosa membrane may require a radical diathermy excision of the lower part of the urethra.

Vulvectomy

Simple vulvectomy may be required, though rarely, for intractable leukoplakia or lichen sclerosus.

Radical vulvectomy is performed for malignant disease of the vulva. It involves a wide dissection of both labia major, labia minor, the lower third of vagina, a wide crescent of suprapubic skin and all the lymph glands draining the area.

Laparoscopy

Space is made in the peritoneal cavity by inflating the abdominal cavity through a blunt ended Verres needle with carbon dioxide to displace the bowel.

The woman is tipped head down the let the intestines slide into the upper abdomen. A laparoscope with a fibreglass light source is now inserted through a hollow trocar permitting examination of the abdominal contents, including the pelvic organs.

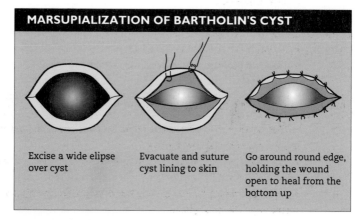

MARSUPIALIZATION OF BARTHOLIN'S CYST

Excise a wide elipse over cyst

Evacuate and suture cyst lining to skin

Go around round edge, holding the wound open to heal from the bottom up

Fig. 23.1 Marsupialization of a Bartholin's cyst.

Laparoscopy may be used for diagnosis of conditions including:
- pelvic inflammatory disease;
- tubal patency;
- endometriosis;
- ectopic pregnancy.

    Treatment may also be carried out through the laparoscope.
- Pelvic adhesions may be divided.
- Deposits of endometriosis cauterized by use of diathermy.
- Small ovarian cysts can be punctured.
- Unruptured ectopic pregnancies can be released.
- Laparoscopic sterilization is performed by applying clips or rings to the tubes. The tubes used to be cauterized with diathermy, but this is less commonly done because of the risks of burning other tissue such as the bowel.

Colpoperioneorrhaphy

This is a posterior vaginal wall repair. It is the repair of a cystocoel and may be combined with vaginal hysterectomy.

Vaginal hysterectomy

Vaginal hysterectomy with or without repair may be chosen if a hysterectomy is indicated and there is also a need to treat prolapse. Usually the uterus should not be greatly enlarged, but it can be done if uterine fibroids are not too large. It may be performed in some cases of cervical intraepithelial neoplasia (CIN).

    The Schauta operation is a radical hysterectomy performed by the vaginal route.

Fistulae

Fistulae may be dealt with through the vagina including a vesico-vaginal or urethral-vaginal fistula provided neither is caused by malignant disease. Some surgeons prefer to repair a vesico-vaginal fistula by opening the bladder through an abdominal incision. A recto-vaginal fistula may also be repaired, although in some cases of intractable fistula a temporary colostomy is needed to allow healing.

    Fistulae associated with malignancy generally require diversion of the urine or colostomy; colpocleisis when the vagina is obliterated is a possible alternative.

ABDOMINAL OPERATIONS

Hysterectomy

When performed by the abdominal route, it may be:

- subtotal hysterectomy;
- total hysterectomy;
- hysterectomy with bilateral salpingo-oophorectomy;
- extended hysterectomy;
- Wertheim's hysterectomy (Fig. 23.2).

SUBTOTAL HYSTERECTOMY

The body of the uterus is removed and the cervix is left. Some believe the cervix and its mucus secretions have an important part to play in sexual function. Its retention may help female orgasm. It certainly is a much easier operation with less risk of ureter damage.

TOTAL HYSTERECTOMY

The whole uterus and cervix is removed and this is now preferred for benign conditions, for the cervix is not left as a possible site for carcinoma. Indications for total hysterectomy include:

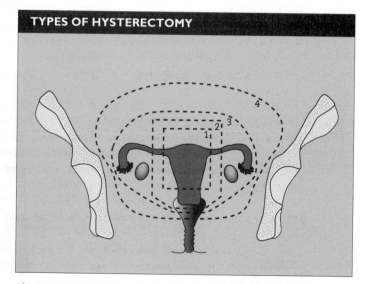

TYPES OF HYSTERECTOMY

Fig. 23.2 Extent of various hysterectomies (see text). 1. Subtotal hysterectomy. 2. Total hysterectomy. 3. Total hysterectomy and bilateral salpingo-oophorectomy. 4. Wertheim's radical hysterectomy.

- fibroids;
- adenomyosis;
- menorrhagia;
- dysfunctional bleeding;
- carcinoma *in situ* of the cervix.

HYSTERECTOMY WITH BILATERAL SALPINGO-OOPHORECTOMY

The removal of the uterus with both tubes and ovaries. The modern tendency is to conserve normal ovarian tissue whenever possible in benign conditions, especially if the woman is still menstruating. Ovarian removal at the time of hysterectomy does prevent ovarian carcinoma, but at the price of the sudden jettison of a major source of oestrogen production in the pre-menopausal woman. The operation may not be feasible if there is chronic sepsis or advanced endometriosis. Both ovaries and the uterus are generally removed in malignant tumours of the ovaries.

EXTENDED HYSTERECTOMY

The operation of choice for carcinoma of the endometrium. It consists in the total removal of the uterus, both tubes and ovaries and a cuff of the vagina; the regional lymph nodes may also be removed if the growth is in the lower third of the uterine cavity.

WERTHEIM'S RADICAL ABDOMINAL HYSTERECTOMY

Performed for carcinoma of the cervix. It consists of the removal of the uterus, tubes, ovaries, broad ligaments, parametria, the upper half of the vagina and the regional lymph nodes.

Myomectomy

This operation involves removal of uterine fibroids with conservation of the uterus. At the abdominal operation, the fibroids are shelled out and the uterus repaired. It is possible to remove large or numerous fibroids and conserve the uterus.

Ventrosuspension

Corrects retroversion of the uterus. It may be achieved by intra-peritoneal shortening of the round ligaments.

OPERATIONS ON THE FALLOPIAN TUBES

Salpingectomy

Removal of the tubes may be partial or total.
- Partial:
  (a) sterilization;
  (b) treatment of ectopic pregnancy.
- Total:
  (a) the whole tube is removed for conditions such as chronic sepsis, tuberculosis and malignant disease;
  (b) total *bilateral salpingectomy* for disease such as chronic sepsis may be combined with hysterectomy as symptoms may persist if the uterus is left.

Other operations

Tubal surgery may be performed to open tubes closed by sepsis or to reverse sterilization. The results for fertility are on the whole disappointing although the use of microsurgery has led to improved results, especially when the tubes have not been diseased before or after sterilization.

Salpingostomy is performed for occlusion of the abdominal ostium. The tube is opened, the fimbriae exposed and a cuff is turned back and sutured in position. When the isthmus and the uterine end of the tube are blocked the tube is divided and either rejoined or *implanted into the uterus*. These methods may be used for reversal of sterilization.

Salpingolysis is the freeing up of a tethered tube by division of peritubal adhesions.

OPERATIONS ON THE OVARIES

Oophorectomy is removal of the whole ovary. It is indicated when all ovarian tissue has been destroyed, for advanced infection and malignant tumours.

At *ovarian cystectomy*, benign tumours or cysts are usually dissected out and normal ovarian tissue conserved and repaired.

Wedge resection for polycystic ovary disease had a vogue, but is now rarely done as alternative treatments are preferred. Multiple punctures of the ovarian capsule have replaced wedge resection.

Cysts of the broad ligament are enucleated from between the layers of the broad ligament.

RADICAL OPERATIONS

Pelvic malignant disease needs resection of the affected organ and the hinterland to which tumour metastases may have been carried.

Lymphadenectomy may be performed when a primary malignant growth is of the cervix and lower uterus. It is usually done after radiation.

Pelvic exenteration is done in cases of advanced carcinoma when no other treatment is possible and the patient is in reasonably good general condition.

Anterior exenteration diverts the urine by implanting the ureters into an ileal loop or into the pelvic colon. The uterus, tubes, ovaries, parametria, vagina, bladder and urethra, together with the pelvic lymph nodes are removed.

Posterior exenteration involves a preliminary colostomy followed by removal of the uterus, tubes, ovaries, posterior vaginal wall, descending colon, rectum and anal canal.

In *total exenteration* the two operations are combined leaving the patient with an ileal loop and a colostomy.

APPENDICECTOMY

Some surgeons used to remove the appendix when opening the abdomen for a gynaecological operation despite the transverse incision making the approach to the caecum difficult in many women. There is a small risk of peritonitis so it is best avoided when performing clean operations such as myomectomy unless the appendix is diseased.

PRE-OPERATIVE PREPARATION

The practice in Great Britain used to be to admit the day before to hospital for gynaecological operations. Recently there has been an increasing use of day case surgery for minor operations such as curettage, termination of pregnancy, laparoscopy and sterilization, so that in some units a third to a half of gynaecological operations are done as day cases.

This has proved popular with women, especially those with children who prefer not to remain in hospital overnight.

The patient should be prepared for operation and the anaesthetic; she must be warned that she may have to remain in hospital if unexpected difficulties arise. Written consent is probably best obtained before the day of the operation in the out-patients or pre-operative assessment clinic. It is essential that a responsible person should accompany the patient to her home.

Clinical examination

HISTORY

A complete history is taken with special attention to any recent illness. The date of the last period should be noted; some surgeons try to avoid major operations in the premenstrual phase when the pelvic organs are more vascular. Examination of the endometrium on the other hand often gives more information if carried out during that time. The possibility of pregnancy should not be ignored. Drugs and medicines recently taken should be noted—these will include hormones, especially oral contraceptives, antibiotics and tranquillizers.

EXAMINATION

A general examination is made. The teeth are inspected and septic lesions in the mouth or throat excluded. The heart and lungs are examined and blood pressure measured. Examination of the abdomen and pelvis follows. The legs are inspected for varicosities.

INVESTIGATIONS

Investigations include an examination of haemoglobin. Except in an emergency, it is unwise to carry out major surgery with a haemoglobin level below 10.5 g/dl, or minor surgery below 10 g/dl. In women of Black origin, a test for haemoglobinopathies is essential.

The blood group and rhesus factor are determined and serum saved in the laboratory. If there is a probability that transfusion will be needed during the operation, the necessary quantity of blood is cross-matched in readiness.

A cervical smear should be examined if it has not been done in the recent past. The urine is tested for albumin and sugar. If there is a suspicion of a urinary infection, a mid-stream sample is sent for bacteriological examination. Renal function tests are advisable if there is a suspicion of abnormal kidney function.

An X-ray of the chest may be taken if indicated. Urography is done before operations when the ureters may be involved, as in Wertheim's hysterectomy to exclude double ureters and other variations. An electrocardiograph is advisable in patients with any suggestion of heart disease. Other investigations may be suggested by the examination or the nature of the case.

Preparation

The patient should be weighed on admission or in the out-patient clinic.

Shaving of the vulva has now generally been abandoned for minor cases although some surgeons prefer it for major vulval and vaginal surgery. Elaborate preparation of the skin is now considered unnecessary, but any septic lesions should be noted and treated. The patient should take a bath and put on a clean operation gown. Cases of prolapse with ulceration of the vagina or cervix will require pre-operative treatment with packs soaked in a suitable antiseptic. In postmenopausal women, pre-operative treatment with oestrogen is helpful; this may be given before admission in the form of oestrogen by mouth or vaginal cream. Antibodies or flagyl may be given before elective surgery.

A light and palatable diet should be given though nothing should be taken by mouth for at least four hours before the operation. The lower bowel should be emptied by a suitable laxative, but enemas and ritual purgation are now little used. If the operation may involve the intestines or rectum, the bowel is emptied and prepared by the use of succinyl sulphathiazole, neomycin or another suitable preparation.

A physiotherapist should visit every patient ideally before the operation and certainly everyone for major surgery. He or she can teach breathing and leg movements for the post-operative period.

Valid consent must be given in writing for the operation by the patient herself. This must be clearly and legibly countersigned by a doctor, who should have explained the operation and its possible sequelae. Girls aged 16 or over sign consent for the operation on their own behalf; for those under that age, the consent of a parent or legal guardian is usually necessary except in an emergency. There may be difficulty in the case of a girl under 16 requesting a termination of pregnancy and insisting that her parents are not to be informed. In such a case, the doctor will have to exercise discretion and act in what he or she considers to be the girl's best interest.

At the time that consent for the operation is obtained, an explanation should be given of the procedure which is contemplated, its nature and effects. In the case of a married woman, her husband's consent is not legally necessary in the UK for operations which lead to sterility such as hysterectomy or sterilization, but it is important that counselling of the couple takes place. It should be made clear in the case of operations for sterilization or vasectomy that the operation should be considered irreversible; on the other hand it must be emphasized that a few failures occur with sterilizations. This advice should be recorded in the case notes.

Counselling in general is important since many women do not understand the anatomy of their pelvic organs and have unnecessary fears concerning the effects of operations, in particular their effects on sexual function. Explanation, if necessary illustrated by a model or diagram, will help to dispel these fears.

POST-OPERATIVE CARE

A period of recovery is required after any surgical operation. After *minor operations* such as dilatation and curettage, the patient can go home on the same day. She should not drive or operate machinery for two days after general anaesthetic. She must be warned to expect some bleeding for up to 14 days after the operation and to abstain from intercourse during that time. More profuse bleeding can follow deep cauterization or conization of the cervix; this may on some occasions be enough to require readmission and possible suture of the cervix.

After *major surgery* such as uncomplicated hysterectomy or prolapse repair, patients are encouraged to get up from bed and move about on the day following operation. Breathing exercises and leg movements are begun from the day after the operation. The length of stay in hospital varies but many can leave after three to six days. Before departure a clear explanation of the operation and the prognosis must be given by a doctor. An adequate period of convalescence at home is necessary before returning to work and normal activity.

The patient may be examined six weeks after the operation. She must be encouraged to return to normal life. Intercourse may be resumed as soon as the vagina is healed. If the ovaries have been removed in the pre-menopausal, the woman should be offered oestrogens by tablet, patch or implant. Patients treated for carcinoma must be followed-up fully.

POST-OPERATIVE COMPLICATIONS

During the first 12 hours after an operation, the patient must be carefully observed for the following:
- respiratory failure or obstruction to the airways;
- shock;
- haemorrhage;
- cardiac failure.

She should be nursed in a recovery unit until she has recovered consciousness and only then returned to a general ward. The pulse rate and blood pressure should be taken and charted every quarter of an hour for the first two hours and thereafter every few hours for the first 12 hours, longer if there is any anxiety.

Pain must be relieved by adequate doses of analgesics such as morphine or pethidine. Patient-controlled analgesia with the woman controlling the flow of weak solutions of analgesia intravenously, is very useful for recovery from elective gynaecological surgery. Addition of promazine or chlorpromazine increases the effect of analgesics and helps to prevent post-operative vomiting.

HAEMORRHAGE

Primary, occurring during the operation and requiring immediate transfusion.

Delayed, occurring during the immediate post-operative period is generally due to a slipped ligature or a bleeding vessel in the vagina or cervix. Blood transfusion is given and the patient returned to the operating theatre to deal with the haemorrhage.

Secondary, occurring up to 14 days after operations and generally from the vagina or cervix, but occasionally from the abdominal wound. Infection is commonly associated, but suture of the bleeding area and blood transfusion still may be needed in all but the slightest cases. After cauterization of the cervix there is generally some bleeding about the 10th and 12th day and patients should be warned to expect this.

Anaemia is common after gynaecological operations and should be prevented with a correct diet.

RESPIRATORY TRACT

Complications of a general anaesthetic include sore throat, tracheitis, bronchitis, bronchopneumonia and massive collapse of the lungs. Breathing exercises should be given after general anaesthetics. Pulmonary infection should be treated with antibiotics. Chest symptoms after the first week sometimes indicate pulmonary embolism.

URINARY TRACT

Retention of urine is common after gynaecological operations and it may be complete or partial. Complete retention of urine often occurs after hysterectomy or repair of prolapse. Rarely hysterical retention occurs after a minor operation such as dilatation and curettage.

Treatment is by immediate catheterization usually emptying the bladder once. If it must be repeated, an indwelling catheter has to be put in for a few days. Some surgeons prefer suprapubic catheterization.

Partial retention of urine is common after operations for prolapse and a catheter should be passed for residual urine five days after operation. Catheter drainage should continue until the residual urine is below 200 ml.

Cystitis and pyelonephritis are very common after gynaecological operations. A catheter specimen or a mid-stream specimen should be examined for evidence of infection after all major operations and suitable treatment given.

Suppression of urine may be due to obstruction to the ureters which may be accidentally injured, ligated or obstructed by a haematoma; it may also be reflex blockage. Warning is often given by unilateral loin ache and a slight temperature. It is a very serious complication and must be dealt with urgently if necessary with relieving surgery by a urologist.

Incontinence of urine through the urethra sometimes occurs after catheterization and in elderly women; it is usually transient. Persistent incontinence suggests a fistula. Urinary fistulae may be vesico-vaginal or uretero-vaginal. These may be caused by trauma at operation, by haematoma formation or by difficult obstetric delivery. They also result from malignant disease.

An uretero-vaginal fistula may follow operations, especially Wertheim's hysterectomy where the ureters are extensively dissected so that their blood supply is imperilled and they become devascularized.

VENOUS THROMBOSIS

Two types can occur after surgery.

Phlebothrombosis is primary venous thrombosis and generally begins in the deep veins of the calf; predisposing causes are:

* trauma;
* anaemia;
* stasis;
* high oestrogen levels.

Thrombophlebitis is caused by infection, generally in the pelvic veins initially and spreading to involve the iliac veins.

Pulmonary embolism can follow thrombosis and if massive is rapidly fatal. Small emboli cause pulmonary infarction.

Prevention of thrombosis and embolism consists of:

* the use of pneumatic boots and leggings during the surgery;
* elasticated stockings worn before, during and after operation;
* early movement;
* avoidance of anaemia;
* prompt treatment of infection;
* prophylactic low dose heparin before and just after surgery.

The contraceptive pill should ideally be stopped six weeks before major elective surgery.

In established thrombosis, heparin is given initially intravenously in a continuous dose of 1000–1500 iu per hour or by separate intravenous injections of 10000 iu every six or eight hours. Calcium heparin can be given subcutaneously. Dindevan (phenindione) is given by mouth and its effect begins in 24 hours. The initial dose is 200 mg, then 100 mg, then 50 mg daily, depending on the prothrombin time, which should be kept at 20 to 30% of normal. Warfarin is an alternative: 30 to 50 mg is given on the first day, none on the second day, then the dose is adjusted according to the International Normalized Ratio (INR) which is a measure of the amount of thromboplastin required to normalize the patient's prothrombin time.

CHAPTER 24

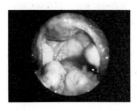

Gynaecological epidemiology

Mortality and morbidity, 291

Benign gynaecological diseases, 292

Hospital episode statistics (HES), 292

GP data on gynaecological conditions, 294

Malignant gynaecological conditions, 295

Carcinoma of the body of the uterus, 297

Carcinoma of the ovary, 297

Gynaecological cancer mortality rates, 298

Sexually transmitted diseases, 298

Termination of pregnancy, 299

Conclusions, 302

Epidemiology started as the statistics of epidemics of infectious diseases. Now the subject is concerned with the study of disease occurrence in populations by comparing prevalence trends, hoping to identify aetiology and means of prevention. More recently in the Western world, epidemiology is involved in Health Service Research and Development.

MORTALITY AND MORBIDITY

This century, life expectancy of women has lengthened over a period of 25 years. In the UK in 1993 it was 79 years of age compared with 74 years in 1960 and 52 at the beginning of the century. Life expectancy is longer in females than in males.

Mortality is not the only indicator of women's health; morbidity has a different pattern between the sexes as well as being higher amongst women than men. Among women there are increased rates of:
- visits to GPs;
- hospital admissions;
- days in hospital;
- days lost from work from acute conditions.

Males have higher mortality rates from some causes of death (coronary thrombosis and cancer), but women have higher rates from infectious, respiratory and digestive conditions. They also have diseases associated with childbearing and the reproductive organs.

Mortality varies with age, being 0.6 per 1000 in girls under 16 and 148.8 in 85 year old women (Fig. 24.1). Further, married women have a

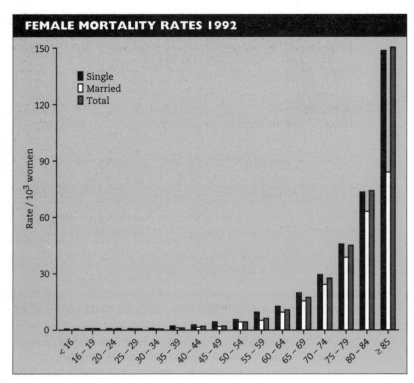

Fig. 24.1 Death rates of women by age.

higher mortality rate than single women (6.2 compared with 3.4 per 1000 in the population). They have higher standard mortality rates in:

- diabetes;
- cerebro-vascular haemorrhage;
- diseases of the liver and pancreas.

BENIGN GYNAECOLOGICAL DISEASES

Hospital episode statistics (HES)

Benign gynaecological conditions are rarely fatal and so mortality rates are not helpful. Hospital episode statistics (HES) are now used as a measure of discharges and deaths from hospitals, but there are problems.

I The analysis of day cases is separate and some analyses do not include them. This means that the gynaecological load is under-analysed, for up

ADMISSIONS AND BED DAYS IN ENGLAND 1991/92

Condition	Ordinary admission	Bed days
Carcinoma of the cervix	10038	87648
Carcinoma in situ	12666	61869
Carcinoma of the body	7793	76786
Benign conditions of the uterus	21871	173961
Benign conditions of the ovary	3187	32428
Hysterectomy	71560	581307
Repair of prolapse	18261	147435
Appendicectomy	44611	201858
Excision of tonsils	72948	167471

Table 24.1 Admissions and bed days in England 1991/92. From Hospital Episode Statistics (Compiled from HES 1994).

to half of women with gynaecological conditions now are treated as day cases.

2 Episodes are counted of hospital care, not people, so if a woman is admitted twice with the same condition, she is counted twice.

Table 24.1 shows the admissions of certain gynaecological conditions and, at the bottom, for appendicectomy and excision of tonsils for comparison. There were about 10000 admissions in 1991/92 for carcinoma of the cervix and the women stayed in for 87000 days, so the average length of stay was 8.7 days. Admissions for carcinoma of the body of the uterus were fewer (7793), but the hospital stay was about 10 days, there being more women in the older age groups. The benign uterine conditions were mostly fibroids and 22000 women with these were admitted with a stay of about eight days on average. Benign conditions of the ovary accounted for 3000 admissions with a stay of about 10 days.

These admission rates fit with the known malignant incidences (see later in the chapter), but these data are the only index we have of hospital work on benign conditions. Turning to operations, 71000 women had a hysterectomy with a stay of about 8.5 days on average, whilst repair of prolapse was the diagnosis for 18000 with an approximate seven days stay.

These data are compared with appendicectomy at 45000 and tonsillectomy at 73000 admissions in the year.

Data like these will be used in the planning of health services and for performance indicators. On their own they are inappropriate units to use

PATIENT CONTACTS AND CONSULTATIONS IN UK

Condition	Age 0–4	5–15	16–24	25–44	45–64	65+
Ectopic pregnancy	0	1	11	11	0	0
Spontaneous miscarriage	0	71	65	1	0	0
Menopausal problems	0	0	1	293	2219	627
Pelvic inflammatory disease	103	65	204	217	113	224
Carcinoma of the cervix	0	0	0	3	5	16
Carcinoma of the ovary	2	3	1	1	11	23
Screening carcinoma of the cervix	0	6	1045	1331	918	181
Contraception	0	138	4707	2559	147	0
Epilepsy	33	48	103	99	78	240
Cholelithiasis	0	7	16	32	28	0

Table 24.2 Patient contacts and consultations in 60 practices of general practice in the UK, September 1991–August 1992. Rate per 10000 patients at risk.

for individual surgeons or hospitals. Some surgeons take more difficult cases; other features are:

- the patient's age;
- social circumstances.

Day case work should be analysed separately in order to give a more complete picture of gynaecological workload.

GP data on gynaecological conditions

The Royal College of General Practitioners and the Office of Population Censuses and Surveys (OPCS) established a group of 60 practices in the UK where details of patient visits were kept, based on symptoms and the general practitioner's opinion of diagnosis. Such GP data are the only national measures of morbidity in gynaecological problems we can get in primary care. Sixty practices provided details on 502493 patients from September 1991 to August 1992.

In Table 24.2, some gynaecological conditions are outlined and, for comparison, epilepsy and gallstone problems are put at the bottom. Students spend a lot of time in medical school learning about epilepsy and gallstones, but it is probable that screening for cervical disease and contraception do not receive anything like the emphasis that is going to be needed in later professional life.

The malignant diseases in gynaecology obviously do not present very often in the average general practice and a practitioner with 2000 patients on his list may expect to see two cases of carcinoma of the cervix and four of carcinoma of the ovary in a year. Two women with ectopic pregnancy would be seen by mathematical chance in that time and 13 spontaneous miscarriages. Thirty women would consult the practitioner about menopausal conditions; this is a subject about which many have little real knowledge of aetiology or modern management. The practitioner might see 90 women with pelvic inflammatory disease in the year, an ill-understood condition, particularly in the very young and those over 65.

The shifts in patient consultations with the general practitioner between 1981 and 1991 in gynaecology were mostly in:

- genito-urinary diseases (increase of 31%);
- urogenital candidiasis (increase of 103%);
- menopausal and postmenopausal conditions (increase of 154% in consultations in the decade).

MALIGNANT GYNAECOLOGICAL CONDITIONS

Cancer Registries collect data about every new case of malignant disease diagnosed in that catchment population (usually the old Regional Health Authority). Data come from:

- hospital in-patient statistics;
- pathology registers;
- radiotherapy registers;
- oncological out-patient clinics;
- colposcopy clinics.

Registries also get death certificates of all cancer deaths in their population, so giving a measure of the total incidence of gynaecological cancer. Mortality rates of malignant disease come from death certificates and are published by the OPCS. Thus there are two distinct sources of epidemiological data about malignant disease:

- the living—prevalence and incidence rates;
- the dead—mortality rates.

In 1990, three gynaecological cancers featured amongst the 10 most frequent cancers among females. Some 4919 women were reported with new cases of carcinoma of the ovary, 3972 with invasive carcinoma of the cervix and 3308 with carcinoma of the body of the uterus. Thus, carcinoma of the ovary has overtaken that of the cervix in the last 20 years as the commonest gynaecological cancer. In 1973 registrations for cervix and ovary were respectively 4065 and 3819.

In the same time period, the deaths reported of the same three cancers were 3995, 1781 and 914. No precise mathematical ratios can be

STANDARDIZED REGISTRATION RATES

Year	Ovary	Endometrium	Cervix
1978	101	100	99
1979	100	100	100
1980	102	101	101
1981	102	100	103
1982	102	100	101
1983	104	96	100
1984	103	96	105
1985	100	96	101
1986	103	98	102
1987	112	94	100

Table 24.3 Trends in registration rates— Standardized Registration Ratio (1979 = 100).

FIVE YEAR SURVIVAL RATE

Condition	Five year survival rates (%)
Carcinoma of the ovary	20
Carcinoma of the endometrium	64
Carcinoma of the cervix	54

Table 24.4 Five-year survival rates for gynaecological cancer in the UK.

derived for the data are of different populations in time—three quarters, half and a quarter, an indication of the poor prognosis of cancer of the ovary compared with that in the cervix; over the years this has worsened for cancer of the ovary and improved for that of the uterus (Table 24.3). The five year follow-up data is in Table 24.4. These differences may represent:

- a real change in the prevalence of a condition;
- a more complete reporting system;
- better diagnostic facilities for making a diagnosis.

The standardized mortality rates (SMR) for carcinoma of the cervix in the following regions of the UK in 1991 were:

	SMR
England	98
Wales	135
Scotland	106
Northern Ireland	81

As the UK has an apparently uniform National Health Service, it is strange to find Wales with a mortality rate about 60% higher than Northern Ireland. This might be due to:

- differences in the socio-economic background of the population;
- differences in the reporting facilities;
- differences in treatment.

There is a trend of increasing incidence of cervical cancer in younger women. So far, there are too few to influence the total statistics, but if there are any specifically increased mortality rate increases, this could cause an increase in the mortality rate for cervical cancer of about 15% by the turn of the century. However, if further *call and recall* screening services for cervical cytology are properly implemented by then, this prediction would be altered.

The geographical incidence of carcinoma of the cervix was highest in Central and Southern America, decreasing as it crossed Europe and Africa to Asia and the Far East. This apparent trend no longer exists. There are many local variations; for example, Portugal has a very high rate of carcinoma of the cervix while its close neighbour, Spain, has a very low one, yet their economic and social characteristics are very similar.

Carcinoma of the body of the uterus

This is unusual under 40 years; incidence rates increase to 55 after which there is a plateau. Increased rates are also found in women who:

- are nulliparous;
- have a late menopause.

There is a reduction in those who have used combined oral contraception.

Carcinoma of the ovary

The ovary is multi-tissue organ. The age of specific incidence rises from 35 to a plateau in the 60s. Rates are higher in Europe and North America than in the rest of the world. This might be due to:

- a difference in the environment;
- a difference in sexual habits;
- a difference in parity;
- increasing longevity;
- better reporting facilities.

Ovarian cancer incidence is decreased with increased completed family size, possibly due to a break in the monthly ovulation pattern with its repeated trauma to the genital epithelium. This is confirmed by the relative risk being decreased with the increasing duration of oral contraception.

Gynaecological cancer mortality rates

Table 24.3 shows the standardized registration rates of women dying in 1991 of three major gynaecological malignancies, Table 24.4 the five-year follow-up of the diseases. Such rates cannot be compared directly with incidence rates for the latter takes place many years before the former. Five-year survival rates after treatment may be a slightly more precise measure. Since cervical carcinoma may recur up to 10 years, a longer time interval than five years may be required. The 15-year survival rate is currently about 30%. There are few recurrences of carcinoma of the endometrium after five years and so that index is a reasonable one; one can say that about two-thirds of women with endometrial cancer are cured.

The survival rate of carcinoma of the ovary is poor and probably reflects are fact that only about a fifth of diagnosed patients are cured. It may be in the future that with more drastic surgery and chemotherapy, this might be improved, but it is still mostly due to late diagnosis of the pathological stage of the disease.

Subdividing these coarse five-year survival rates into stages gives a better idea of the problem. For example, in the UK most carcinoma of the cervix is either Stage I or Stage II when diagnosed compared with developing countries when it is either Stage III or even IV.

Good epidemiological data is collected nationally on some gynaecological conditions—examples from the Genito-Urinary Medicine (GUM) clinics and recognized centres performing legal abortions.

SEXUALLY TRANSMITTED DISEASES

The treatment of sexually transmitted diseases (STD) in the UK is mostly in special (GUM) clinics. These are required to make returns on the number of cases seen each quarter to the Department of Health. The data are not quite so precise as they first appear. There may be over-reporting for the returns are of patients' visits, not of individual patients who could attend several times at the same or even different clinics. There is no mechanism for record linkage.

Conversely, there also may be under-reporting because GUM clinics do not treat all cases of STDs. An unrecorded number may be treated in:
• general practice;
• private sector;
• gynaecological clinics;
• antenatal clinics.

Despite this, data collection on STD in the UK is better than most countries in the world.

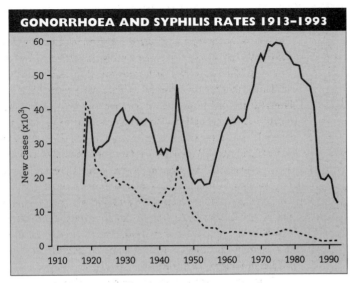

Fig. 24.2 Incidence of gonorrhoea (—) and syphilis (---) in England 1918–93.

The prevalence of different STD has changed due to the alterations in treating the diseases and the new antibiotics. Figure 24.2 shows the alterations in two major diseases since 1910. Syphilis rates have declined since the time of the First World War with a slight peak at the time of the Second World War, but since has continued decreasing. Gonorrhoea, which had its apex in 1975, is diminishing greatly. Age specific rates, however, show that gonorrhoea is increasing in the under 16s and the over 35s. The commonest notified disease now is non-specific urethritis, which is more of a male problem.

The change in sexual attitudes has occurred mostly in the young who have more frequent and multi-partnered intercourse. Non-barrier contraceptives, such as the oral contraceptive, aid in the spread of infection, but the advent of HIV has altered sexual and contraceptive habits with more barrier methods being used.

TERMINATION OF PREGNANCY

Induced abortion is legal on certain grounds in England, Wales and Scotland, but not in Northern Ireland. If two doctors consider the risk to the mother or fetus of certain events to be greater if the pregnancy continued rather than if it were stopped, they can recommend termination of pregnancy. This is dealt with in Chapter 20.

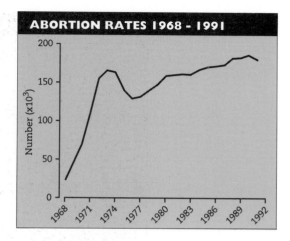

Fig. 24.3 Total number of abortions in England and Wales 1968–91.

Data on legal termination of pregnancy are collected by the Department of Health and published by the OPCS every year. In 1991 there were 179522 legal abortions in England and Wales of which 167326 were for residents of those countries.

The number of abortions rose sharply with the passing of the Abortion Act in 1967 but increased more steadily in the last thirteen years (Fig. 24.3). There has actually been a decline in number since 1989.

Terminations for non-residents has fallen considerably with other European countries and the USA now having more liberal Abortion Acts. The main source of non-residents in 1991 was France (2486) and Ireland (Eire 4154 & Northern Ireland 1775).

Figure 24.4 shows age specific abortion rates. By far the greatest group are the 20 to 30 year olds. At the two ends of reproductive life terminations of pregnancy are more readily performed, but there are not so many represented in the data.

Table 24.5 shows that some 86% of terminations took place before 13 weeks and only 1.8% after 20 weeks. The numbers tail off enormously after 22 weeks for after this time it is virtually only the late diagnoses with congenital abnormalities that are an indication.

In 1991 a change was made to the Abortion Act so that whilst 24 weeks was considered the earliest viability, this timing only applied to the indications relating to maternal health and life. The congenital abnormalities indication was timeless and so termination of pregnancy could in theory take place right up to full gestation, although this would not happen very often.

Among resident women having termination of pregnancy, 77523

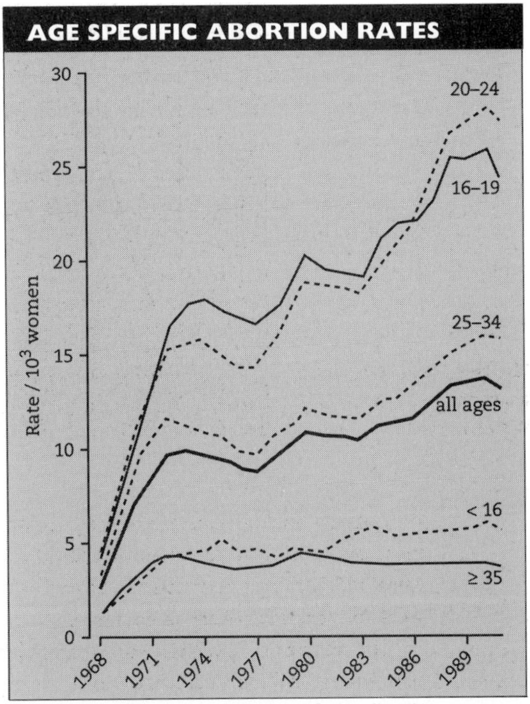

AGE SPECIFIC ABORTION RATES

Fig. 24.4 Age specific abortion rates. Residents of England and Wales 1968–1991.

GESTATIONAL AGE AT TERMINATION

Gestation (weeks)	Number	%
<9	62310	35.0
9–12	92222	51.2
13–19	21621	12.0
>20	3369	1.8

Table 24.5 Gestational age at termination of pregnancy, 1989–1991.

(66%) were single. Under half the terminations (57618–43%) were performed in NHS units, the rest in the private sector. This might be because:

• there are insufficient facilities in the NHS;
• the woman might wish to go privately because she wants the privacy;
• the NHS Trusts are buying private beds because it may be cheaper to do this than run the service themselves;
• there are agencies such as the British Pregnancy Advisory Service that are subsidising terminations.

CONCLUSIONS

Using epidemiology, we can look at trends geographically, in time and related to patients' background characteristics. This allows us to tease out aetiology and to predict needs. Data should be collected at all hospitals and should be used by departments at their audit meetings and in their hospital reports. Eventually one can tie this to cost benefit and correctly based performance indicators will be determined.

Index

Page references in *italic* type refer to figures, and those in **bold** type refer to tables.

abdominal distension 267
abdominal examination 4–5
  auscultation 5
  deep palpation 4
  light palpation 4
  percussion 4
  scars *5*
abnormal uterine bleeding 122–3
  intermittent bleeding 122–3
  menstrual variations 122
abortion 241–7
  criminal 190–1, 255
  early 244–5
    complications 244
    future pregnancies 244–5
  epidemiology 299, *300, 301*
  late 245
  menstrual extraction 246–7
  methods 243–4
  mid-trimester 245–6
    complications 245–6
    hysterotomy 245
    morcellation and extraction 245
    prostaglandins 245
  septic 254–5
  therapeutic 247
  UK position 241–3
  see also miscarriage
Abortion Act 1991 242
acquired immuno-deficiency syndrome 147–9
acute abdomen 265–75
  checklist 270
  diagnosis 267–9
    examination 267–8
    history 267
    investigations 268–9
  distension 267
  nausea and vomiting 266–7
  out of pregnancy
    endometriosis 272
    ovarian tumour 271–2
    pyosalpinx 271
    salpingitis 270–1
    torsion of fallopian tube 271
    uterine fibroids 269–70
    vaginal trauma 269
  pain 265–6
  in pregnancy
    abortion 272
    appendicitis 274–5
    bowel problems 275
    ectopic pregnancy 273
    pyelonephritis 274
    rectus haematoma 275
    red degeneration of fibroid 273
    retroverted uterus 272–3
    round ligament stretch 274
  shock 266
adeno-acanthoma of vulva 62
adenomyosis 87–8
  differential diagnosis 88
  pathology 87
  signs 88
  surgery 88
  symptoms 87–8
  treatment 88
adreno-genital syndrome 45
AIDS 147–9
amenorrhoea 116–22
  genital agenesis 116
  primary 116–18
    causes 116
    investigation 117
    management 117–18
    treatment 116
  secondary 118–22
    causes 118–20
      general disease 119–20
      physiology 118
      pituitary 118–19
      psychology 118
      thyroid disease 119
      uterine 119
    investigation 120–1
      history 120
      physical examination 120
      tests 120–1
    treatment 121–2
anatomy 15–46
  bladder 32
  congenital malformations 41, *42–3*
  embryology of pelvic organs 38, *39–40, 41*
  fallopian tube *19–21*
  ovary 15, *16–18*
  pelvic arterial blood supply *33, 34*
  pelvic diaphragm 28, *29–31*
  pelvic lymphatic drainage 35–6
  pelvic nerve supply *36–8*

anatomy (*cont.*):
  pelvic venous drainage *34, 35*
  ureter 31–2
  urethra 32
  uterus 20, *21–6*
    relations 24
    structure *22, 23*
    supports 25–6
  vagina 26–7
  vulva 27–8
androblastoma 110
androgenital syndrome 118
annulment of marriage 191
anorgasmia 189
anovulation, causes of 194
anterior exenteration 284
anvil uterus 41
appendicectomy 284
appendicitis 274–5
arcuate uterus 41
artificial insemination 206–7
  disclosure of donor 207
  donors 206
  HIV 206–7
  samples 206
  technique 207
atrophic vaginitis 68–9
auscultation 5
Ayre's spatula *211*

barium enema 13
barrier contraception 229–30
Bartholin's glands 28
  cyst removal *279*
  swellings of 59–60
basal cell carcinoma of vulva 63
basal temperature charts *198*
bicornuate uterus 42
bimanual examination 6
bivalve speculum 6, 7
bladder, anatomy 32
blood, investigations 8–9
bowel
  endometriosis of 152
  history 3
  problems in pregnancy 275
Brenner tumour 108

carcinoid tumour 109
carcinoma
  cervix 73–9
  embryonal 108
  endometrial 88–90
  fallopian tube 101
  intra-epithelial 63
  mortality rates 298
  ovarian 110–14
  screening for 209–16
    cervix 209–15
      benefits of cervical screening 215
      current position 209–10
      effectiveness of cervical screening

213, *214–15*
      examination of smear 212–13
      grading smears 213
      taking smear 210, *211–12*
    ovary 216
  urethral 60
  uterine 88–90
  vulva 63
  see also *individual cancer types*
cervical cancer see cervix, cancer of
cervical circlage 257
cervical erosion 71–3
  acquired 72
  congenital 72
  diagnosis 72
  symptoms 72
  treatment 72–3
cervical interepithelial neoplasia 75–6
  treatment 76
cervical polyp 73
cervical secretions, improvement of 200
cervical smear test 209–15
  benefits of cervical screening 215
  current position 209–10
  effectiveness of cervical screening 213,
    214–15
  examination of smear 212–13
  grading smears 213
  taking smear 210, *211–12*
cervicitis 71–3
  acute 71
  cervical erosion 71–3
    acquired 72
    congenital 72
    diagnosis 72
    symptoms 72
    treatment 72–3
  chronic 71
cervix 71–9
  anatomy 24
  cancer of 73–9
    aetiology 73
    cervical interepithelial neoplasia 75–6
      treatment 76
    diagnosis 75
      ancillary methods of 75
      differential 75
    pathology 74
    physical signs 74
    screening see cervical smear test
    staging 75
    symptoms 74
    treatment 76–9
      complications of 79
      palliative 79
      pelvic exenteration 78
      radiotherapy 77
      results of 78
      surgery 77, *78*
    urinary frequency 74
cervical polyp 73
cervicitis 71–3
  acute 71
  cervical erosion 71–3

acquired 72
  congenital 72
  diagnosis 72
  symptoms 72
  treatment 72–3
  chronic 71
  lymphatic drainage 35
chancroid 150
chemical contraceptives 230–1
chemotherapy
  ovarian carcinoma 113–14
  vulval carcinoma 62
Chiari-Frommel syndrome 118
chlamydia 144
chorioadenoma destruens 262
chorioncarcinoma 91, 263
chromosome defects 43–6
  adreno-genital syndrome 45
  Klinefelter's syndrome 44–5
  non-disjunction 43
  sexual identity 45
  super females 44
  testicular feminization 45
  true hermaphrodites 45
  Turner's syndrome 44
  virilization 46
clip sterilization 237
clitoris 28
  hypertrophy 59
coital difficulties, correction of 200
coitus interruptus 231
colpoperioneorrhaphy 280
colpotomy 278
complications of early pregnancy 249–63
  chorioadenoma destruens 262
  chorioncarcinoma 263
  ectopic pregnancy 257–61
    causes 258
    clinical features 259
    differential diagnosis 260
    incidence 258
    investigations 259–60
    pathology 258–9
    treatment 260–1
  hydatidiform mole 261–2
    clinical features 261
    follow-up 262
    incidence 261
    investigations 261
    treatment 261–2
  miscarriage 249
    causes of 249–52
      fetal 250–1
      incidence of 251–2
      maternal 249–50
      parental compatibility 251
    clinical features and management 252–7
      complete miscarriage 253
      counselling 256–7
      criminal abortion 254
      incomplete miscarriage 253
      inevitable miscarriage 252–3
      missed abortion 253–4

  recurrent abortion 255–6, 257
  septic abortion 254–5
  threatened miscarriage 252
computerized tomography 12
condylomata acuminata 59
condylomata lata 59
congenital malformations 41–3
  fallopian tubes 41, 93
  and miscarriage 251
  ovary 41, 103
  uterus 81, 82
contraception 217–32
  barrier methods 229, 230
  chemical contraceptives 230–1
  coitus interruptus 231
  counselling 218–19
  douching 231
  injectable contraceptives 225
  intrauterine devices 224–9
    advantages 226
    complications 227–8
    contra-indications 228
    disadvantages 226–7
    method of insertion 228–9
    post coital contraception 229
    pregnancy 229
  methods used by both partners 220
  methods used by female 219–20
  methods used by male 220
  oral contraceptives 220–5
    combined pill 220–4
      advantages 220
      contra-indications 222–3
      drug interactions 223
      forgotten pills 224
      metabolic effects 220, 222
      prescribing of 223–4
      side-effects 222
    emergency pill 224
    progestogen-only pill 224–5
  safe period 231, **232**
  sheath 231
  trends in 217–18
corpus luteum cysts 106
crab lice 57
criminal abortion 190–1
crossed hostility test 197
cryotherapy 129
curettage 129
Cusco's speculum 6, 7
cystocoele 164
cystometry 177
cysts, of vulva 59
cytology 9–10

dermoid teratoma 108–9
detrusor instability 175
  treatment 178, 179
dilatation and curettage 277–8
douching 231
drug sensitivity, and pruritus vulvae 57
Duck Bill speculum 6, 7
duplex uterus 42

Dutch cap 229, *230*
dysgerminoma 108
dysmenorrhoea 130–2
　secondary, congestive or acquired 132
　spasmodic 130–1
　　cause 131
　　management 131
dyspareunia
　deep 188
　superficial 187–8

ectopic pregnancy 97–101, 257–61
　and acute abdomen 273
　causes 97, 258
　clinical features 98, 259
　differential diagnosis 260
　incidence 97, 258
　investigations 259–60
　pathology 98, 258–9
　ruptured 99, *100–1*
　　diagnosis 100
　　treatment 100–1
　treatment 260–1
　unruptured 98, 99
ejaculatory failure 184–5
embryonal carcinoma 108
endodermal sinus tumour 108
endometrial carcinoma 88–90
　aetiology 88
　investigations 89
　pathology 89
　signs 89
　staging 89, 90
　symptoms 89
　treatment 89–90
endometriosis 151–8
　and acute abdomen 272
　classification 152, **156**
　definition 151–3
　diagnosis 153–7
　　differential 155–7
　pathology 151–2
　physical signs 155
　sites of 152–3
　　abdominal wall 152
　　bowel 152
　　ovaries 152
　　pelvic peritoneum 152
　　perineum and vagina 152
　　urinary tract 152
　　uterine ligaments 152
　stages of *154–5*
　symptoms 153, *154–5*
　treatment 157–8
　　hormone therapy 157–8
　　surgery 158
endometritis 82
endometrium
　examination of infertility 198–9
　histology 10
　menstrual cycle 52
enterocoele 164
epidemiology 291–302

benign gynaecological diseases 292–5
　GP data 294–5
　hospital episode statistics 292, **293**,
　　294
　gynaecological cancer mortality rates
　　298
　malignant gynaecological conditions 295,
　　296–7
　mortality and morbidity 291, *292*
　sexually transmitted diseases 298, *299*
　termination of pregnancy 299, *300*, *301*
erectile dysfunction 186–7
examination 4–8
external genitalia, embryology 39, *40*
external urethral meatus 28

fallopian tubes 93–101
　anatomy *19–21*
　benign tumours of 101
　carcinoma of 101
　congenital malformations 41, 93
　ectopic pregnancy 97–101
　　causes 97
　　clinical features 98
　　incidence 97
　　pathology 98
　　ruptured 99, *100–1*
　　　diagnosis 100
　　　treatment 100–1
　　unruptured 98, 99
　embryology *39*
　lesions of 200–2
　nerve supply 35
　patency 199
　pelvic thrombophlebitis 97
　physiology *55*
　relations *19*, 20
　salpingitis 93
　　acute 94–5
　　　abdominal examination 94
　　　clinical features 94
　　　differential diagnosis 94–5
　　　investigations 94
　　　treatment 95
　　　vaginal examination 94
　　chronic 95
　　tuberculous 96
　structure 19–20
　surgery 283
　torsion of 93, 271
family history 3
Ferguson's speculum 6
fibroadenoma 107
fibroids 83–7
　and acute abdomen 269–7
　aetiology 84
　degeneration 85
　diagnosis 85
　　differential 86
　effects on childbearing 86–7
　investigations 85
　pathology *84*–5
　red degeneration of 273

surgery 86, *87*
  symptoms 85
  treatment 86
follicular cysts of ovary 105–6
follicular maturation *16*
follicular stimulating hormones 50, *51*
foreign bodies in vagina 69
fungal infection, vulva 57

gamete intra-fallopian tube transfer (GIFT)
    205
gardnerella 65–6
  investigations 65–6
  symptoms and signs 65
  treatment 66
genital prolapse
  classification 162, *163–4*
  differential diagnosis 165–6
  physical signs 165
  prevention 166
  symptoms 164–5
  treatment
    palliative 166–7
    pessaries *167–8*
    physiotherapy *168*
    post-operative care 170–1
    pre-operative care 169–70
    prognosis for future pregnancies 171
    surgery 169
  uterine 60, 164
germ cell tumours 108
germ cells 48
germinal inclusion cysts 106
GIFT 205
glycosuria, and pruritus vulvae 58
gonadoblastoma 109
gonorrhoea 144–6
  investigations 145
  symptoms and signs 145
  treatment 145–6
Graafian follicle *17*
Grafenberg ring 225
granuloma inguinae 149–50
granulosa cell tumour 109

haemorrhage 288
haemorrhagic cysts of ovary 106
hermaphroditism 45–6
history taking 1–3
HIV 147–9
Hodge pessary 161, *162*, *163*
hormones
  investigations 10
  in treatment of endometriosis 157–8
hot flushes 136
human immuno-deficiency virus (HIV)
    147–9
  investigations 148–9
  symptoms and signs 148
  treatment 149
hydatidiform mole 261–2
  clinical features 261

follow-up 262
  incidence 261
  investigations 261
  treatment 261–2
hymen 28
hymenectomy 278
hypomenorrhoea 122
hysterectomy 129–30, 281–2
  with bilateral salpingo-oophorectomy
    282
  extended 282
  subtotal 281
  total 281–2
  vaginal 280
  Wertheim's 282
hysterotomy 245

imaging 10–13
  barium enema 13
  computerized tomography 12
  intravenous urography 13
  magnetic resonance imaging 11, *12*
  pelvic lymphangiography 13
  ultrasound 10, *11*
  X-rays 12
in vitro fertilization 204–6
  artificial insemination 206–7
  direct injection of sperm into oocyte
    206
  gamete intra-fallopian tube transfer
    (GIFT) 205
  in utero injection (IUI) 206
  indications for 204
  results 205
  technique 204–5
  zygote intra-fallopian transfer (ZIFT) 206
incontinence see urinary incontinence
infection
  ovary 104
  urinary tract 180
  uterus 82–3
  vagina 63–5
  vulva 57
infertility 193–207
  adoption 207
  assisted fertilization 204–7
    artificial insemination 206–7
      disclosure of donor 207
      donors 206
      HIV risk 206–7
      samples 206
      technique 207
    direct injection of sperm into oocyte
      206
    gamete intra-fallopian tube transfer
      (GIFT) 205
    results 205
    technique 204–5
    in utero injection (IUI) 206
    zygote intra-fallopian transfer (ZIFT)
      206
  causes of anovulation 194
  causes of sterility 193–4

infertility (*cont.*):
  investigation of infertile couple 194–9
    examination of female 195
    examination of male 195
    female history 194–5
    investigations 195–9
      basal temperature charts *198*
      examination of endometrium 198–9
      hormone tests 199
      post coital test 195–6
      seminal analysis 196–7
      sperm antibodies *197*
      tests for tubal patency 199
      ultrasound 199
    male history 195
  treatment 199–202
    correction of coital difficulties 200
    improvement of cervical secretions 200
    lesions of tubes 200–2
    lesions of uterine body 200
    sperm hostility 200
    male infertility 202–4
inguinal hernia 60
injectable contraceptives 225
internal iliac artery 33, *34*
intra-epithelial carcinoma 63
intrauterine devices 225, *226*, 227–9
  advantages 226
  complications 227–8
  contra-indications 228
  disadvantages 226–7
  method of insertion *228–9*
  post coital contraception 229
  pregnancy 229
intravenous urography 13
invasive mole 262
investigations 8–13
  urine 9
iron deficiency anaemia, and pruritus vulvae 58
Irving operation *235*

Klinefelter's syndrome 44–5

labia major 28
labia minor 28
  hypertrophy 59
laparoscopy 279–80
leukoplakia, of vulva 58
lichen sclerosus et atrophius 58
Lippes loop 225, *226*
luteinizing hormone 50–1
lymphadenectomy 284
lymphogranuloma venerum 150

Macdonald suture *257*
magnetic resonance imaging 11, *12*
males
  sexual problems 184–7

ejaculatory failure 184–5
erectile dysfunction 186–7
premature ejaculation 185–6
sterility
  causes of 193
  treatment of 202–4
malignant melanoma of vulva 63
menopause 135–42
  continued periods 140–1
  physiology 135–7
  postmenopausal bleeding 133–4
  postmenopausal therapy 137–40
    complications of 140
    hormone replacement 137, *138–9*
      preparations 139
    long-term 139–40
  premature 121, 141–2
    cause 141
    management 141–2
    treatment 142
  symptoms 136–7
    dry vagina 136
    genital changes 136–7
    hot flushes 136
    long-term 137
menorrhagia 123–30
  aetiology 123–4
  clinical course 124–5
  treatment 125–30
    diagnosis 125, *126, 127*
    drug therapy 126–8
    hormonal 128
    non-hormonal 128
    surgical therapy 129–30
menstrual extraction 246–7
menstruation 53
  disorders of 115–34
    abnormal uterine bleeding 122–3
    amenorrhoea 116–22
      genital agenesis 116
      primary 116–18
      secondary 118–22
    dysmenorrhoea 130–2
      secondary, congestive or acquired 132
      spasmodic 130–1
    menorrhagia 123–30
      aetiology 123–4
      clinical course 124–5
      treatment 125, *126, 127*–30
    postmenopausal bleeding 133–4
    premenstrual tension 132–3
  history 2
  menstrual cycle 51, *52*–3
  menstrual flow 53–4
  menstrual loss *54*
mesonephroma 108
metro-menorrhagia 122
metrorrhagia 122
micturition, history 2–3
miscarriage 249
  and acute abdomen 272
  causes of 249–52

fetal 250–1
  incidence of 251–2
  maternal 249–50
  parental compatibility 251
clinical features and management 252–7
  complete miscarriage 253
  counselling 256–7
  criminal abortion 255
  incomplete miscarriage 253
  inevitable miscarriage 252–3
  missed abortion 253–4
  recurrent abortion 255–6, 257
  septic abortion 254–5
  threatened miscarriage 252
  see also abortion
molluscum contagiosum 59
monilia 67–8
  symptoms 67–8
  treatment 68
mons 28
morcellation and extraction 245
mortality and morbidity 291, 292
mucinous cystadenoma 107
Mullerian ducts, failure of fusion 41, 42, 81, 82
Multiload-cu 375 227
musculature, pelvic diaphragm 29, 30, 31
myomectomy 282

nausea and vomiting 266–7
nocturnal enuresis 181
Novagard 227

obstetric history 2
oestrogens 49–50
oral contraceptives 220–5
  combined pill 220–4
    advantages 220
    contra-indications 222–3
    forgotten pills 224
    metabolic effects 220, 222
    prescribing of 223–4
    side-effects 222
  emergency pill 224
Orthogyne-T 227
ovarian artery 33
  surgery 283
ovary 103–14
  anatomy 15, 16, 17–18
  benign tumours
    androblastoma 110
    Brenner tumour 108
    carcinoid tumour 109
    dermoid teratoma 108–9
    fibroadenoma 107
    germ cell tumours 108
    gonadoblastoma 109
    granulosa cell tumour 109
    mesonephroma 108
    mucinous cystadenoma 107
    pseudomyxoma peritonei 107

serous cystadenoma 106–7
    solid teratoma 109
    thecoma 110
  carcinoma of 110–14
    and acute abdomen 271–2
    chemotherapy 113–14
    epidemiology 297
    metastatic 111–12
    parovarian tumour 112
    in pregnancy 114
    screening for 216
    spread 110–11
    staging 111
    treatment 112–13
  congenital malformations 41, 103
  cysts 105–6
    corpus luteum 106
    follicular 105–6
    germinal inclusion 106
    haemorrhagic 106
    theca lutein 106
  diagnosis 104–5
    examination 104–5
    history 104
    investigations 105
    symptoms 104
  embryology 38
  endometriosis 152
  infections 104
  ovarian hormones see individual hormones
  physiology 47, 48
  relations 18
  structure 15, 16, 17–18
overflow incontinence 175–6
  treatment 179–80

parental compatibility, and miscarriage 251
parovarian tumour 112
pelvic blood supply
  arterial 33, 34
  venous drainage 34
pelvic diaphragm 28, 29–31
pelvic examination 5–6
pelvic exenteration 78, 284
pelvic fascia 29
pelvic lymphangiography 13
pelvic lymphatic drainage 35–6
pelvic nerve supply 36, 37–8
pelvic pain 265–6
pelvic peritoneum, endometriosis 152
pelvic thrombophlebitis 97
perineal body 30
perineotomy 278
perineum, endometriosis 153
pessaries 167–8
  Hodge 161, 162, 163
  ring 167
physiology 47–56
  fallopian tube 55
  menstruation 53
    measurement of menstrual loss 54
    menstrual cycle 51, 52–3

menstrual flow 53–4
physiology (*cont.*):
  organ function 51–4
  ovarian hormones 49–51
    oestrogen *49–50*
    pituitary gonadotrophin hormones 50,
      51
    progesterone 50
  ovary 47, *48*
  uterus 51
  vulva and vagina 56
polycystic ovary syndrome 122
polymenorrhoea 122
polypi
  cervical 73
  uterine 83
Pomeroy operation *234*
post coital contraception
  hormonal 224
  intrauterine device 229
post coital test 195–6
posterior exenteration 284
postmenopausal bleeding 133–4
pregnancy
  early, complications of see complications
      of early pregnancy
  and intrauterine devices 229
  ovarian tumours in 114
  and prolapse repair 171
  termination see abortion
premature ejaculation 185–6
premenstrual tension 132–3
  aetiology 132–3
  symptoms and signs 132
  treatment 133
progesterone 50
progestogen-only pill 224
prolapse 162–71
prostaglandins, and mid-trimester abortion
    245
pruritus vulvae 57–9
  causes 57–8
  investigations 58
  treatment 58–9
pseudomyxoma peritonei 107
pudendal arteries 34
pudendal nerve *37*
pulmonary embolism 289
pyelonephritis 274
pyometra 82–3
pyosalpinx 271

radiotherapy
  cervical cancer 77
  squamous epithelioma of vulva 62
rape 190
rectal examination 8
rectus haematoma 275
reflex incontinence 176
respiratory complications of surgery 288
retroversion of uterus 159–62
  and acute abdomen 272–3
  causes 159, *160–1*

diagnosis 161
  symptoms 161
  treatment 161, *162*
round ligament stretch 274

safe period 231, **232**
salpingectomy 283
salpingitis 93
  acute 94–5
    abdominal examination 94
    clinical features 94
    differential diagnosis 94–5
    investigations 94
    treatment 95
    vaginal examination 94
  and acute abdomen 270–1
  chronic 95
  tuberculous 96
salpingolysis 201
salpingostomy 201
sarcoma 90
scabies 57
seminal analysis 196–7
septate uterus 42
septic shock syndrome 68
serous cystadenoma 106–7
sexual identity 45, 46
sexual problems 183–91
  annulment of marriage 191
  criminal abortion 190–1
  females 187–9
    anorgasmia 189
    deep dyspareunia 188
    superficial dyspareunia 187–8
    vaginismus 188–9
  history and examination 183–4
  males 184–7
    ejaculatory failure 184–5
    erectile dysfunction 186–7
    premature ejaculation 185–6
  rape 190
sexually transmitted diseases 143–50
  chancroid 150
  chlamydia 144
  epidemiology 298, *299*
  gonorrhoea 144, *145–6*
  granuloma inguinae 149–50
  human immuno-deficiency virus 147,
      148–9
  lymphogranuloma venerum 150
  syphilis 146–7
sheath (condom) 231
Sheehan's syndrome 118
Shirodkar suture *257*
shock 266
silastic ring sterilization 237, *238*
Simmond's disease 118
Sim's retractor 6, *7*
social history 3
solid teratoma 109
speculum 6, *7*
sperm antibodies *197*
sperm hostility 200

squamous epithelioma of vulva 61, 62
  chemotherapy 62
  clinical features 61
  differential diagnosis 61
  methods of spread 61
  pathology 61
  radiotherapy 62
  treatment 61–2
sterilization 233–40
  clip 237
  counselling for 233
  female 233–9
    causes of failure 238–9
    laparoscopic 235, 236, 237, 238
    laparotomy 234, 235
    Irving operation 235
    male 239–40
    Pomeroy operation 234
    silastic ring 237, 238
  stress incontinence 174–5
    treatment 177, 178
subseptate uterus 42
super females 44
surgery 277–90
  adenomyosis 88
  appendicectomy 284
  cervical cancer 77, 78
  endometriosis 158
  fallopian tubes 283
  fibroids 86, 87
  hysterectomy 281–2
  ovaries 283
  post-operative care 287
  post-operative complications 287–9
    haemorrhage 288
    respiratory tract 288
    urinary tract 288–9
    venous thrombosis 289–90
  pre-operative preparation 284–7
    clinical examination 285
    preparation 285–7
  radical operations 284
  transcervical ablation 128–9
  vaginal and vulval operations 277–80
    colpoperioneorrhaphy 280
    colpotomy 278
    dilatation and curettage 277–8
    hymenectomy 278
    laparoscopy 279–80
    perineotomy 278
    vaginal hysterectomy 280
    vulvectomy 279
syphilis 146–7
  investigations 146
  symptoms and signs 146
  treatment 147

termination of pregnancy see abortion
testicular feminization 45, 118
theca lutein cysts 106
thecoma 110
thrombophlebitis 289
thrush see monilia

thyroid disease, and amenorrhoea 119
torsion of fallopian tube 93
total exenteration 284
transcervical ablation 128–9
trichomonas 66–7
  investigations 66–7
  symptoms and signs 66
  treatment 67
tuberculous salpingitis 96
Turner's syndrome 44
  and amenorrhoea 118

ultrasound 10, 11
  in infertility 199
unstable bladder 178–9
ureter, anatomy 31–2
urethra
  anatomy 32
  carcinoma of 60
  dislocation of 164
  examination 6
  prolapse 60
  urethral caruncle 60
urinary fistula 174
urinary frequency 180–1
urinary incontinence 174–6
  detrusor instability 175
  overflow incontinence 175–6
  reflex incontinence 176
  stress incontinence 174–5
  treatment
    overflow incontinence 179
    stress incontinence 177, 178
    unstable bladder 178, 179
  urinary fistula 174
  urodynamic investigation 176, 177
urinary tract
  endometriosis 153
  infection 180
  surgical complications 288–9
urine, investigations 9
urogynaecology 173–81
  nocturnal enuresis 181
  physiology 173
  urinary frequency 180–1
  urinary incontinence 174–6
    detrusor instability 175
    overflow incontinence 175–6
    reflex incontinence 176
    stress incontinence 174–5
    treatment 177–9
      overflow incontinence 179
      stress incontinence 177, 178
      unstable bladder 178, 179
    urinary fistula 174
    urodynamic investigation 176, 177
  urinary tract infection 180
uterine artery 33–4
uterus 81–92
  abnormal uterine bleeding 122–3
    intermittent bleeding 122–3
    menstrual variations 122
  adenomyosis 87–8

differential diagnosis 88
uterus (cont.):
  pathology 87
  signs 88
  surgery 88
  symptoms 87–8
  treatment 88
  anatomy 20, 21–6
    ligamentous supports 25–6
    structure 22, 23–4
  chorioncarcinoma 91
  congenital malformations 41, 81, 82
  embryology 39
  endometrial carcinoma 88–90
    aetiology 88
    epidemiology 297
    investigations 89
    pathology 89
    signs 89
    staging 89, 90
    symptoms 89
    treatment 89–90
  endometrial polypi 83
  fibroids 83–7
    aetiology 84
    degeneration 85
    diagnosis 85
      differential 86
    effects on childbearing 86–7
    investigations 85
    surgery 86, 87
    symptoms 85
    treatment 86
  infections 82–3
    endometritis 82
    pyometra 82–3
  inversion 60
  lymphatic drainage 35
  mixed mesodermal tumours 90–1
  nerve supply 35–6
  pathology 84–5
  physiology 51
  prolapse 60, 164
    see also genital prolapse
  retroversion 159–62
    causes 159, 160–1
    diagnosis 161
    symptoms 161
    treatment 161–2
  sarcoma 90
  uterine ligaments, endometriosis 152
uterus didelphys 42

vagina 63–9
  anatomy 26–7
  changes in
    childbirth 56
    sexual activity 56
  congenital malformations 42–3
  dryness 136

embryology 39, 40
endometriosis 153
examination 5
foreign bodies in 69
infections of 63–5
  examination 64–5
  investigation of partner 65
  investigations 65
  symptoms 64
  treatment 65
lymphatic drainage 35
microbiology 65–9
  atrophic vaginitis 68–9
  gardnerella 65–6
  monilia 67–8
  septic shock syndrome 68
  trichomonas 66–7
physiology 56
relations 27
structure 26–7
vaginal artery 34
vaginal cones 168
vaginal diaphragm 229, 230
vaginal discharge 2, 57, 64, 72
vaginal trauma 269
vaginismus 188–9
varicose veins, of vulva 59
venous thrombosis 289–90
ventrosuspension 282
vestibule 28
virilization 46
vitamin deficiency, and pruritus vulvae 58
vulva 57–63
  anatomy 27–8
  embryology 39, 40
  examination 5
  lump in 59–60
  lymphatic drainage 35–6
  malignant disease of 61–3
    adeno-acanthoma 62
    basal cell carcinoma 63
    intra-epithelial carcinoma 63
    malignant melanoma 63
    squamous epithelioma 61, 62
  physiology 56
  pruritus vulvae 57–9
    causes 57–8
    investigations 58
    treatment 58–9
  radical vulvectomy 62
  varicose veins 59
vulvectomy 279

Wertheim's radical hysterectomy 77, 78

X-rays 12

ZIFT 206
zygote intra-fallopian transfer (ZIFT) 206